How to use natural cures
to reverse respiratory ailments

The

Respiratory Solution

Finally, relief from
asthma, bronchitis, mold,
sinus attacks, allergies,
sore throats, colds and flu

Dr. Cass Ingram

Knowledge House
Buffalo Grove, Illinois

Disclaimer: This book is not intended as a substitute for medical
diagnosis or treatment. Anyone who has a serious disease should
consult a physician before initiating any change in treatment or
before beginning any new treatment.

For ordering information call (800) 243-5242 or for overseas
orders call (847)-473-4700. To send a fax: (847) 473-4780. To
send an e-mail: droregano@aol.com. For more information about
the products mentioned in this book see the Web site, Oregacyn.com.

ISBN: 1-931078-02-5

Table of Contents

Introduction

Respiratory diseases are one of the most common of all medical conditions. It seems that virtually everyone suffers from some type of respiratory complaint. Sinus problems, colds, flu, sore throat, scratchy throat, irritable nose, runny nose, itchy eyes, allergies, shortness of breath, asthma, hay fever, ear ache: everyone occasionally suffers from one or more of these conditions.

Today, respiratory problems are an international epidemic. Yearly, significant outbreaks happen all over the world. The incidence of asthma, bronchitis, persistent cough, pneumonia, sinusitis, and emphysema is increasing astronomically. Even whooping cough has made a comeback.

Respiratory illnesses are a vast dilemma: billions are affected not just yearly but also monthly, perhaps daily. However, there is no need to suffer endlessly from such conditions. There is a cure, and the cure comes from nature. In contrast, drugs fail to cure respiratory illnesses. Natural medicines are capable of curing them, because they greatly aid the function of the lungs. What's more, there are a number of natural substances, which, if taken regularly, may prevent the occurrence of lung or respiratory diseases.

In order to comprehend why respiratory infections are so common the function of the lungs must be reviewed. The lungs are a reactionary system. They sort the good from the bad, the healthy from the toxic, and the clean from the filthy. They are a type of living filter system with the ability to expunge anything undesirable. This means they are able to cleanse the air to a large degree before it enters the lungs and, therefore, the blood. If that cleansing function fails, disease develops. Other parts of the respiratory tree, such as the tonsils and nostrils, also perform this function.

When the lungs become overwhelmed as a result of the inhalation of toxins, germs, or other debris, the result is inflammation. The toxins in fact activate the lung's immune system, leading to swelling and inflammation. This may result in difficulty breathing, mucous build-up, and/or cough. The swelling and inflammation, if unresolved, breeds further infection, because congestion of the tissues aids in microbial growth.

The lungs are the largest organs in the respiratory system, and they are the primary ones involved in respiratory diseases. Other respiratory organs include the throat (trachea), bronchial passages, sinuses, nasal passages, mouth, and ear canals.

Today, there is a greater vulnerability for the development of diseases of the lungs and other respiratory organs than ever before in history. The air we breathe is never clean. It is so heavily polluted that lung damage is inevitable. In fact, in the Western world in particular no one can escape. Thus, there is extensive air pollution in every city and every corner of the globe. Obviously, some regions are more polluted than others, the worst being major metropolitan areas, like Los Angeles, New York City, Chicago, Rome, Istanbul, Cairo, Tokyo, or

Athens. Yet, no region is pollution free, so no one on this globe escapes the toxic effects of noxious air.

Global warming aggravates the dilemma. A hot atmosphere accelerates the toxicity of airborne pollutants. Plus, dry weather increases the level of toxic particles, since rain is needed to flush them from the air. Thus, in drought-like conditions air quality worsens significantly.

Deforestation also increases the risks for respiratory pollution. Trees are the primary means for removal of noxious carbonic gases, like carbon dioxide and carbon monoxide, from the atmosphere. Carbonic gases are categorically respiratory poisons. What's more, the destruction of the rain forest has accelerated the release of certain germs into the atmosphere. For instance, currently, across the globe mold counts are at the highest level ever recorded.

The question is how can the lungs and other organs be protected from this toxicity? What foods, supplements, vitamins, minerals, and herbs offer significant protection? Plus, which herbs or plant extracts are potent enough to halt respiratory symptoms and/or reverse disease? These are the questions which will be thoroughly answered by this book.

The respiratory system is a combination of organs, which function as a unit. It includes the lungs, bronchial tubes, throat, sinuses, mouth, and even the ear canals. Of course, the lungs are the largest and most significant component. These organs have a vast surface area and, thus, act as a potential breeding ground for germs.

Complaints of the respiratory system are the main reason people see doctors. There are hundreds of respiratory conditions, some minor and some serious. A partial list of these conditions includes colds, flu, croup (in children), asthma, bronchitis, pneumonia, pleurisy, congestive heart failure, sinusitis, post nasal drip, sinus headache, runny nose, laryngitis, hoarseness, sore throat, tonsillitis, emphysema, and ear aches.

Usually, respiratory conditions cause what are merely transitory symptoms. However, if the condition is untreated and/or neglected, a chronic illness may develop. Some respiratory illnesses are lethal: for instance, asthma. In hospitalized patients pneumonia is a major cause of death, particularly for cancer patients and those with suppressed immunity. Emphysema is often fatal, as are certain rather remote lung diseases, like asbestosis, berylliosis, and silicosis.

Cancer is perhaps the most feared of all respiratory illnesses. It is a devastating disease and, once it is diagnosed, it usually results in a rapid death. Cancer may attack any part of the respiratory system, although it most commonly develops in the lungs. However, throat cancer is an epidemic in Westernized countries. In smokers lung cancer is the number one cause of death. However, the consequences can be positive, that is if the individual utilizes natural medicine in concert with medical care. Even with cancer the lungs can heal, that is if they are provided with the proper nutrients and are treated with the appropriate herbal tonics.

There is yet another reason the lungs make us vulnerable: they are the primary portal of entry for a wide range of poisons. They are the most readily accessible of all pathways by which dangerous substances can enter the body. This is because whatever is inhaled deep into the lungs may also readily be absorbed into the general circulation, that is into the blood and lymph. A good example is anthrax. This is a germ which normally causes illnesses, but not fatalities. The fatalities are caused by the biological form of anthrax, the one made by the military-industrial complex. This war-grade anthrax was made specifically to kill and to do so quickly and in vast numbers. If the entire quota of anthrax stored in the U. S. stockpiles was released throughout the continental United States, if unprotected, virtually every North American would die. Anthrax kills through the lungs, in other words, you must breathe it to become seriously sickened.

The likelihood of mass destruction from a rare germ like anthrax is minimal. The more likely cause of epidemics and, therefore, potentially thousands of deaths are more universal germs, like the flu virus. Anthrax, Hantavirus, West Nile virus, and similar rare germs will always cause their share of deaths. However, the more serious epidemics will be caused by germs that are more widespread, like influenza, staph, strep, and fungus. These are everyday germs found everywhere. What's more, they are nearly always found on or in people, continuously. These are the germs of global epidemics that will likely cause the majority of deaths and disabilities in the coming decades.

This is not to underestimate the powers of the more bizarre germs. Untold numbers of lung and respiratory infections are caused by such germs and, thus, their role must always be considered in diagnosing or treating the condition. In fact, all types of germs must be considered in order to properly address the true cause of each illness. For more information about which germs may be involved in a given condition see Chapter 4.

Even so, there is a need to simplify the treatment of respiratory diseases. What is needed are agents which neutralize the major factors which cause such diseases. These factors are germs, allergens, and pollutants. Incredibly, these are the very agents with which an entire category of living creatures must contend every day, that is the plant kingdom. The trees, shrubs, grasses, herbs, and food plants have continuously adapted mechanisms to survive the aforementioned insults. Their mechanism is to produce chemicals, which act to neutralize any toxicity.

Have you ever wondered how plants, such as the trees which line a busy interstate highway, survive despite being constantly exposed to pollutants? They do so by producing special substances known as *phytochemicals*. The purpose of these substances is to help the plants combat stress, including the stress from pollutants as well as germs. Today, it is possible to extract these plant chemicals and use them for personal protection. In the plant kingdom there is a medicine for virtually any illness (a statement originally attributed to the Prophet Muhammad). This is an upbeat view, indicating that if we are ill, we should never lose hope. The challenge is finding the appropriate "medicine" and determining how it should be used. The information in this book helps solve this issue, that is to provide you with the appropriate plant medicines you need to reverse your respiratory complaints and to protect your lungs and other organs from toxic and/or microbial insults.

Chapter 1

The Breathing Mechanism

We breathe, because air is necessary for survival. The oxygen in the air is nourishment for the body. Oxygen is just as important, in fact, it is more important, than food or water. People have lived up to a month without food and a week or more without water. However, without air we can only live a few minutes.

Air is inhaled into the lungs. It eventually reaches the tiny cells, that is the alveoli, located throughout the lung tissue. The alveoli act to deliver the oxygen from the air into the blood. This oxygen is then captured by the red blood cells, which transport it through the blood and ultimately deliver it to the cells.

An old Reader's Digest book, *Our Human Body: its Wonders and Care,* provides an excellent overview of the lungs. J. D. Radcliff notes that human beings subject the lungs to all sorts of insults. For instance, he describes how slumping, sitting in a sloppy manner in soft chairs, cramping the body while sitting, etc., all impair their ability to keep us healthy. Smog, gasoline fumes, car exhaust, cigarette smoke, and industrial chemicals, as well as fumes from household cleaners and pesticides, damage these delicate organs on contact. Incredibly, the lungs are inflated a half billion times in a lifetime, which amounts to a massive amount of strain on such a fine organ system. Obviously, the lungs are more durable than any man-made machine, which could never withstand so many repetitions.

The lungs would go into shock if they were directly and immediately exposed to pollutants or particulate matter as well as to extremes in air temperature. This is solved by the nose, which conditions the air and filters particulate matter. Every breath can have a potentially lethal amount of dust particles as well as allergens and microbes. Here again, the nasal passages and sinuses act as a buffer, filtering noxious items and producing mucous to lubricate, cleanse, trap, and condition. As described in the *Digest* the mucous is a type of sticky compound, which traps any dust that passes over it, much like a warm gluey surface collects dust. Obviously, if all of the dust is trapped, with time this accumulates and could clog the system. However, in its immense miracles the body has its own "street cleaners": the cilia, tiny hair-like projections with their own independent sweeping power, helping to cleanse the tissue linings and mucous of particulate matter.

The lungs have a vast blood supply. This is so that the red blood cells can mix readily with the air. The red cells contain a complex molecule called hemoglobin. It is the hemoglobin which traps oxygen so it can be transported to the cells and organs.

Everyone knows that blood is red. However, in certain areas the blood appears dark blue or purple: the blood inside veins, for instance. This blood is depleted of oxygen. Plus, it is high in carbon dioxide. When the venous blood is returned to the lungs, the oxygen is replenished and carbon dioxide is expelled. In other words oxygen is what makes blood red. That is why the blood of people on oxygen tanks is unusually bright red.

Oxygen is crucial for sustaining health. It is the most vital life force. In contrast, carbon dioxide is a poison. If it accumulates to excess, life ceases. It is crucial that the body receives plenty of oxygen, while removing as much carbon dioxide as possible. The purpose of breathing is to draw in sufficient oxygen and drive out the carbon dioxide. Anything which impairs breathing, such as spinal disease, abdominal illnesses, poor posture, stress, lung disease, antagonistic medications, etc., will diminish health by impairing oxygen intake and increasing carbon dioxide retention.

The lungs are crucial for cleansing the tissues. Exhaled gases contain a wide range of toxins, that is the various waste products from cellular metabolism. *Physiology and Hygiene*, published in 1900, describes this toxicity. The authors note that the waste gases from human exhalation are not only poisonous to the individual, but they are also poisonous to the group. Have you ever noticed a heavy or foul "human smell" in closed rooms with lots of humans? That smell isn't body odor; it is the odor of foul human gases from exhaled air.

It is crucial to have healthy breathing to maintain superior health. In order to do so take deep breaths often and exhale thoroughly. Healthy breathing is an art which must be practiced. Incredibly, we often forget to breathe and rarely take the time to take a deep breath. The fact is relaxed deep breathing is such a powerful technique that it may result in an immediate health improvement.

With every breath there is a trade: oxygen for carbon dioxide and other waste gases. This is what sustains life. If this trade is imbalanced, ill health results. If it stops, so does life.

Yet, to breathe pure oxygen is dangerous, except for very

short periods of time. Pure oxygen would excessively accelerate the metabolic rate, causing the body to essentially burn itself out. Thus, air is naturally a mixture of gases, mainly nitrogen and oxygen with a small amount of carbon dioxide. Normally, the carbon dioxide level in the atmosphere is lower than 1%. However, as a result of pollution the levels are continuously rising. Thus, even the fresh air we breathe is inadequate for optimal health, because the body regards any inhaled carbon dioxide as noxious. Carbon monoxide, the gas resulting from automobile emissions, is even more noxious and is, in fact, a lung and tissue poison. High levels of carbon monoxide in inhaled air can quickly lead to death.

J. C. McKendrick, in *Principles of Physiology*, provides a fascinating overview of the function of the lungs. He claims that breathing allows the excretion of carbon in the form of carbon dioxide. This carbon dioxide is produced as a result of normal cellular activities. All living cells, plant and animal, produce it. This gas is found in various organs as well as the blood and lymph.

The lymph provides the cells with nutrients, but it is also a respiratory organ, closely tied to every breath. Breathing moves lymph, in other words, the lungs act as a sort of heart for the lymphatic system. Every time we breathe, lymph is pumped. The lymph absorbs oxygen from the lungs and delivers it to the cells, which then dump carbon dioxide back into it. Ultimately, the lymphatics dump the carbon dioxide-rich fluid into the blood so it can be disposed of.

Mouth breathing: a source of illness

Few people realize it, but it is dangerous to breathe through the mouth. The mouth is naturally the passage for food. The lungs are the passage for air. Reversing this is abnormal. William Krohn, M.D., author of *Physiology and Hygiene*, claims mouth breathing is "very harmful." He states that air should always be breathed through the lungs, that is through the nostrils. The lungs and bronchial tubes, he says, are designed to receive air, to condition, moisten, and filter it. The nostrils, acting as the smelling organ, help us sense dangerous odors, toxins, and harmful compounds, which may, as a result, be avoided. With mouth breathing no such warning occurs. Thus, mouth breathing may allow us to breath unhealthy air continuously, air which we might have sought to avoid had we used our natural nasal sensor system. Dr. Krohn describes that the person who habitually breathes through the mouth may experience a variety of symptoms, while having no clue that it is due to mouth breathing. Symptoms of mouth breathing include dry throat, colds, stuffy sinuses, stuffy nose, runny nose, and even lung disease. In fact, Dr. Krohn explains that the development of lung disease is a certainty as a result of continuous mouth breathing. Incredibly, he claims that colds can be easily prevented by breaking this habit.

The lungs are the main organs of respiration. All other organs, like the nose, trachea, sinuses, and bronchi, are ancillary. The lungs are arranged in a magnificent manner. Miraculously, they have a massive surface area, allowing the greatest possible exposure for air, that is oxygen, absorption.

Respiration is not just to bring in air: it is also to purify the blood. The fluids in our bodies, the blood and lymph, are formed as a result of digestion. In other words what we eat leads to the creation of the nutritive body fluids. Blood delivers the nutrients from the food to the cells, plus it removes toxins, so they can be excreted. The lymph is also made from food. However, the lymph, which flows towards the heart from the various outer regions of the body, like the limbs, is a waste product. It transports the residues resulting from the degeneration of tissues. Ultimately, the lymph, which resembles a sort of protein-rich cream, is dumped into the bloodstream, and from there it is delivered to the heart.

Like the lymph vessels, the veins carry waste material back toward the heart. The waste laden lymph and venous blood are pumped from the heart into the lungs. Here, these fluids are cleansed and revitalized. Oxygen from the inspired air is the primary cleansing agent.

According to physiology textbooks respiration is defined as the function by which venous blood, that is dark red or bluish-red blood, is converted to arterial blood, that is bright red blood. This, of course, occurs in the lungs and is the result of oxygen. It is also the result of the exhalation of the poisonous carbon dioxide, which is the main agent responsible for the dark color of venous blood. This process of cleansing and detoxifying the blood is absolutely crucial. Any halt in it rapidly results in death, largely because of oxygen deficiency and the accumulation of metabolic poisons. Proper breathing is absolutely crucial for this process. Any restriction in breathing, as well the inhalation of poor quality of air, will lead to an increase in metabolic poisons and, therefore, ill health.

Most people fail to breathe properly. They rarely take the time to take deep breaths. Or, they are under an extreme amount of stress and, thus, their breathing is inhibited or constrained breathing. This perpetuates poor health and may lead to actual disease. To become as healthy as possible improve your breathing habits. Take time to take deep breaths. Find out what you are doing that is impeding or restricting your breathing. Improvement in the breathing process will often result in a dramatic enhancement in health.

The importance of deep breathing

Lung disease is often the result of improper breathing practices. It seems rather incredible; however, some people forget to breath. Others restrict their breathing because of poor posture or stress.

Breathing is an art. It is a form of exercise. Many individuals have conditioned themselves to breath improperly. Thus, it may be necessary to get a breathing coach or buy books which teach proper breathing exercises. A lack of proper breathing curbs the intake of oxygen, the most necessary of all nutrients. A deficiency of oxygen may cause hundreds of symptoms. This may explain the rather sudden improvement people experience just by adopting improved breathing practices.

Sleeping: your position affects your health

The Prophet Muhammad was the first to delineate the importance of sleeping positions. He recommended foremost sleeping on the right side. Here is what he said. First, choose the right side for sleeping, and make every attempt to discipline yourself to do so. If you must have an alternative, try the left side. Avoid sleeping on the back. The worst position, according to the Prophet, was stomach sleeping.

His recommendations are medically sound. Let us review recommendations from a scientific/medical point of view:

"Sleep on the right side." The heart is tucked next to the rib cage on the left side, its tip pointing downward at an angle towards the back of the rib cage. Sleeping on the left side forces the ribs directly against the heart, impairing its ability to pump blood. This causes the heart to work harder, wearing it out more quickly and increasing the risks for heart failure. The aorta, the major tube guiding blood from the heart to the rest of the body, is also on the left side, and left-sided sleeping partially collapses it. Sleeping on the back places tension on all of the spinal muscles, because the flat-back position causes vertebral strain, especially in the lower back. Persistent back sleeping is a major cause of chronic lower back pain. What's more, sleeping on the back creates torque on the lower thoracic and upper lumbar vertebrae. These vertebrae are attached to the diaphragm, the key muscle responsible for breathing. Sleeping on the back greatly strains the diaphragm, making it work exceptionally hard. Back sleeping also compromises the function of the heart. The natural position would be for the heart to lay against the left side of the right lung. Thus, the heart is resting upon soft tissue instead of bone. This allows blood to be pumped without restriction. Thus, sleeping on the right side greatly reduces structural and gravitational stress on the heart and arteries, as is illustrated by the following case history:

Mr. S. suffered from chronic heart failure, which failed to respond to medications. He was placed on a special diet, given osteopathic manipulative treatments (to balance the spine and release restrictions), and told to sleep only on his right side. Within a month he improved dramatically. His cardiac condition was ultimately completely resolved.

Stomach sleeping is the most dangerous of all positions. Such a position completely violates the normal physiology of the body. The lungs must expand. Stomach sleeping is essentially sleeping with the full weight of the body upon them. Obviously, this prevents the lungs from properly functioning. What's more, because of the pressure of the weight of the body against the delicate respiratory tract, stomach sleeping encourages mouth breathing. The fact is stomach sleeping is so dangerous that it may be considered a significant cause of lung and sinus diseases as well as perhaps a cause of premature death.

As an osteopathic physician I observed a number of patients who had damaged their spinal structures, posture, and body conformation, as well as their overall health, through persistent stomach sleeping. Eventually, through a change in position and osteopathic manipulative therapy much of the damage was reversed.

Chapter 2

Where Disease Lurks

Air is supposedly healthy, yet, it can be the most dangerous thing on earth. The air may either nourish and sustain us or sicken and poison us. Gases are among the most poisonous substances known. The wrong kinds of gases can kill more quickly than the most deadly oral poison.

Dangerous air, everywhere

The air in virtually every civilized region is contaminated. Certainly, the air in major North American cities is unfit for breathing. In huge cities, such as Los Angeles, Chicago, New York City, San Diego, San Francisco, and Toronto, it is essentially poisonous.

One study determined that people living in Los Angeles suffer tremendous lung damage. In fact, the majority of residents living in this city for more than ten years suffer from a type of chronic emphysema. This means children living in this region are in essence doomed to suffer permanent lung damage, all the result of environmental contamination.

There are hundreds of pollutants in city air. The majority of these pollutants arise from vehicular exhaust. Industrial exhaust fouls the air with a host of toxins, including mercury, lead, arsenic, cadmium, beryllium, sulfur dioxide, carbon dioxide, carbon monoxide, dioxins, toxic hydrocarbons, and thousands of others. Jet exhaust is an enormous contributor to air pollution. In cities with international airports the air may be so polluted as to be deemed virtually cancerous.

Basement air—unusually dangerous

Avoid basements, especially in strange houses. Go into them only if absolutely necessary. One of the quickest ways to compromise health is to breathe basement air, especially in an individual who is already ill. The exception is basements which have plenty of sunlight or in which fresh air is circulated by opening windows or patio doors. If the basement has no sunlight, then the air may well be deadly. The fact is such basements, devoid of sunlight and ventilation, should have posted at their entrance: Warning: enter at your own risk.

Stagnant basement air is permeated with potentially disease producing germs and noxious gases. The greatest threats are the molds, which thrive in the cold, dark and often moist environment. A great deal of illness could be prevented by simply avoiding entering strange basement environments.

Basements breed disease. The lack of sunlight encourages the growth of a wide range of pathogens, especially molds and fungi. When the lack of sunlight is combined with excessive moisture, the scenario is set for massive mold growth. Merely inhaling this foul air may cause symptoms if not frank illness.

It is important to be aware of how dangerous this air is. This is because millions of individuals develop various symptoms of illness, having no idea it is caused by the air they breath. What's more, basement air is so dangerous that a few inhalations of contaminated air may lead to a lung or sinus infection.

Basement air, filled with mold, poisons and spores, can cause
a wide range of symptoms. A partial list includes:

- sinus attacks
- post nasal drip
- sinus headaches
- neck pain
- rash
- achiness
- pneumonia
- depression
- psychotic behavior
- itchy skin
- cold sensations

- runny nose
- sinus pain
- pain in the head
- neck stiffness
- joint pain
- flu-like symptoms
- chest pain
- agitation
- attention deficit
- itchy scalp
- sore throat

This is an incredibly long and varied list of symptoms, all
due to the inhalation of poisonous, mold-infested air. This fully
illustrates how dangerous the air is in moldy regions. Thus, if
you are exposed to such air, the appropriate precautions must be
taken to avoid serious illnesses if not outright disease. Even cancer has been associated with mold infestation. A low white count
may also be caused by mold poisoning. Obviously, molds have
a dire effect upon the immune and respiratory systems, as is
illustrated by the following case history:

Mr. C. is a 40 year old with a tendency to developing sinus problems. Recently, his basement was flooded, and a number of books and other items were soaked. The water was cleaned out, but after the flood a noticeable odor developed in the basement. He went down to inspect it and detected a foul odor. Soon thereafter he developed severe neck and head pain, the pain in the head being across the occiput (back of the head). He felt cold all over and sluggish. Reasoning that he had developed mold poisoning, he took large amounts of Oreganol (oil of wild oregano) as well as the desiccated spice known as Oregacyn. The symptoms quickly dissipated, and he was free of all pain within two hours. He was very impressed, because when he had developed similar "mold" reactions previously, the symptoms lasted for days or weeks.

Chemical pollutants

The inhalation of noxious chemicals is an enormous cause of disability, ill health, and even death. It is also one of the major causes of lung and throat cancer.

The United States is the most chemically polluted region in the world. Tens of thousands of chemicals are used in industry, agriculture, and home use. The exposure to noxious chemicals is daily. Long term exposure increases the risks for a variety of respiratory diseases, particularly bronchitis, sinusitis, emphysema and cancer.

People in the United States suffer a vast degree of diseases due directly to chemical pollution. Millions of people are sickened yearly due to such toxicity. While there are no medical cures, natural medicines offer great hope for reversing much of this toxicity. This is because natural medicines help the body remove toxic chemicals. Plus, natural compounds act as antioxidants, helping to minimize the toxicity of synthetic chemicals. Herbs, spices, vitamins, minerals, enzymes, amino acids, and essential fatty acids all offer healing actions in reversing or minimizing the toxicity of airborne pollutants. The most powerful herbs and spices include sage, rosemary, cumin, coriander, oregano, and cloves. Anti-pollution vitamins include vitamin A, beta carotene, vitamin C, pantothenic acid, and folic acid. Minerals which fight pollution toxicity include magnesium, zinc, and selenium, with selenium being the most important one. However, spice extracts are the most powerful and rapidly acting of all detoxification agents. They are potent antioxidants, many times more potent than vitamins and minerals. Plus, they kill both molds and fungi as well as noxious bacteria. They also assist the lungs in removing harmful chemicals.

There is little that can be done to reverse the air pollution debacle. For the home environment air purifiers/ionizers may help considerably. However, this illustrates the need to consume protective agents to prevent or reverse lung damage. While the antioxidant and lung-protective powers of certain vitamins are well respected, there are even more powerful substances available. Spice extracts have recently been proven to be the most powerful of all. A recent study (2002) by the USDA found that of all natural antioxidants tested spices were the best. What's more, of all the spices the top was wild oregano. It proved to have some 40 times the antioxidant effect of apples and over five times the action of the well respected antioxidants in blueberries. This clearly illustrates the value of consuming concentrates of wild oregano, such as Oreganol and/or Oregacyn, as agents for reversing and/or preventing pollution-induced lung damage.

Chapter 3

Germs, Germs, Everywhere

The air we breathe is never sterile. Usually, it is teeming with germs. Yet, germs infect the lungs from other sources besides the air. The germs in food and water may also infect them.

The role of parasites

A parasite is an organism that cannot live on its own. It must derive its food, nutrition, and housing from its host. In animals parasitic infection is common and is virtually normal. As described by Hanna Kroeger in her book, *Parasites: the Enemy Within*, humans may house as many as 100 types of parasites. She continues that the danger is that most Americans regard parasitic diseases as a problem in Third World or tropical countries. They fail to understand that currently parasitic infections are an American epidemic and that tens of millions of individuals are afflicted. Certain investigators regard it now to be the norm, that is the majority of North Americans suffer from some degree of infestation.

Parasites are a major cause of lung disease. The lungs are a type of filter, and parasites may be trapped there from the blood. Plus, lung tissue is rich in nutrients, and parasites tend to lodge in nutrient-rich tissue. The lungs are rich in red blood: parasites feed off of it.

Doctors rarely diagnose parasitic lung disease. This is mainly because they rarely consider it as a serious possibility. For instance, an entire book, *Introduction to Respiratory Diseases,* published by the National Tuberculosis and Respiratory Disease Association, fails to mention parasites. Thus, there is a lack of education, as well as awareness, for doctors regarding the importance of these noxious germs in causing acute and chronic lung disorders. The poor rate of diagnosis is also because there are few if any tests that can accurately confirm the presence of these organisms within the lungs. Parasites hide deep within lung tissue and rarely cause any obvious lung signs. In fact, the infection becomes visibly evident only when it is chronic, severe, and massive. What's more, acute parasitic infection is even more rarely diagnosed, largely because doctors fail to consider it. The symptoms mimic more common conditions. In fact, when this infection does strike, it is usually diagnosed as the flu or pneumonia. Yet, if a careful history were taken, there would be a higher degree of suspicion and, therefore, a more rapid resolution of symptoms

If a high level of suspicion became the mainstay, parasitic lung infection would be more commonly discovered. The typical history is as follows: the onset of a rather sudden, severe case of respiratory distress—that is coughing, chest pain, fever, chills, sweating, aches/malaise—combined with the potential exposure to contaminated food or water. A sudden bout of pneumonia in an individual who rarely develops it is another warning. Traveling overseas while eating uncooked food or drinking various cold beverages increases the risks and begs the diagnosis.

Fungal infections

This is perhaps the most under-diagnosed of all lung infections. The majority of doctors are aware of its existence. Yet, often they fail to respect the seriousness of it or how common it truly is. In an individual with a chronic lung condition that fails to respond to traditional treatment, fungal infestation should be seriously considered as the culprit.

Medical texts describe lung fungal infections as "exceedingly common." Exposure to the cause of these infections, that is mold spores, is nearly continuous, especially in warm and/or damp climates. Through the air we breathe these spores readily enter the respiratory tract, lodging in the lungs. They may not immediately cause outright disease, yet, they must always be regarded as a foreign irritant. Yet, under certain circumstances, such as stress, drug therapy, or a weakened immune system, they can grow in a fulminant fashion, causing severe respiratory symptoms. A course or two of antibiotics may provoke such an infection. This is because by destroying the inhibitory healthy bacteria and, thus, altering immunity they encourage the growth of molds and fungi. A wide range of diseases may be caused by mold/fungal infection of the lungs. A partial list includes asthma, chronic or acute bronchitis, pneumonia, sinusitis, ear aches, rhinitis, pleurisy, and pharyngitis.

Molds and fungi readily enter the lungs. To some degree they are filtered out by the nose and sinuses. However, mold spores are relatively small and, thus, can penetrate deep into the lungs. What's more, if the molds or yeasts infect the sinuses, contaminated secretions may drip into the lungs, infecting them as well.

In contrast to parasites there are a number of medical tests which can aid determining the existence of lung fungus. The number of fungi which may infect the respiratory tract are legion and include aspergillus, penicillium, histoplasma, coccidiodes, cryptococcus, nocardia, blastomyces, and actinomyces. Many of these fungi are regional, for instance, coccidiodes is a desert fungus and blastomyces is a river valley fungus. Individuals who visit regions where these fungi are endemic are highly vulnerable to developing the disease, because they have no immunity against it. The fact is the people who live there locally may have the infection chronically and not even be aware of it.

Mold in homes

If you suddenly develop a health problem, particularly lung and/or sinus disorders check for mold in your house. Mold gets into the home in several ways. Symptoms of mold intoxication may vary greatly. A few of the more common symptoms include:

- Joint pain
- Sinus attacks
- Watery eyes
- Itchy eyes
- Itchy nose
- Shortness of breath
- Spastic muscles
- Neck pain
- Spinal stiffness
- Chronic ear infection
- Attacks of sneezing
- Runny nose
- Headaches
- Pain behind the eye
- Chest pain
- Wheezing
- Loss of bladder control
- Dizziness
- Headaches
- Insomnia

- Sudden awakening at night
- Attention deficit
- Forgetfulness
- Anger/frustration
- Confusion
- Lowered energy
- Nausea
- Cough
- Hives
- Scratchy throat
- Exhaustion
- Inability to focus on work
- Bleeding from the lungs
  (coughing up blood)

- Poor concentration
- Mood swings
- Psychotic tendencies
- Irritability
- Apathy
- Bloody nose
- Vomiting
- Allergic reactions
- Sore throat
- Hay fever-like symptoms
- Vague abdominal pain
- Weakness
  - Spots on the lungs
    (visible by X ray)

The role of food allergies

Allergies play an enormous role in lung and respiratory problems. In fact, in many instances they may play the primary role.

I used to be a bronchitis sufferer. Every fall or winter I would get a severe case, which would last for as long as two months. I might endure several episodes per year. Then I learned of the importance of food allergies. Through a sophisticated blood test I discovered my allergenic foods. When I removed those foods from my diet, which included wheat, rye, celery, asparagus, butter, cheddar cheese, perch, and Swiss cheese, the bronchitis disappeared, never again to return.

The bizarre issue is that the aforementioned foods are technically wholesome. Yet, even seemingly healthy foods can be toxic, that is if you are allergic to them. This toxicity damages the immune system, leaving the body vulnerable to the development of various infections as well as diseases.

Allergenic foods have a major impact upon the function and health of the lungs. They cause a significant degree of toxicity, perhaps more than airborne allergens.

Foods contain hundreds of chemicals in the form of various unique molecules, proteins, sugars, and fats. In other words, they are rather complex substances. Certain of these molecules are known to evoke allergic responses. This is one reason certain natural foods may provoke severe reactions. Incredibly, it is possible that something as natural as broccoli or asparagus could provoke severe or chronic allergic reactions. Today, things are even more complex, because foods are heavily processed. Plus, they contain added chemicals. These chemicals are aberrant, that is they are synthetic and unknown to nature. Thus, the immune system usually recognizes them as foreign, that is it regards them as toxic. As a result the immune cells attack the chemicals and/or the food, setting the stage for allergic intolerance. Thus, the body recognizes the food as toxic, because it is infiltrated with synthetic, dangerous chemicals.

Food intolerance is a major cause of respiratory disorders. Ear infections, colds, flu-like symptoms, sore throats, tonsillitis, asthma, sinus, and bronchial conditions may all be primarily due to food allergies. Could a sore throat be caused by food allergies? Indeed, I have seen dozens of cases where the continual consumption of noxious or allergenic foods leads to terrible sore throats. Antibiotics are taken in an attempt to quell the pain and supposed infection, but they are ineffective. Plus, this approach fails to take into account the fact that toxic foods are depressing the immune system. Even strep throat may have in its origin from food allergy, because these allergic reactions deplete the immune reserve, making the throat vulnerable to bacterial invasion.

Just why each individual has his/her own pattern of allergenic foods is largely unknown. Heredity may play a role, as does the individual's dietary habits. Regarding the latter, simply consuming certain foods to excess may result in allergy. In fact, this is one of the most common causes of food allergies. Environmental toxins are another major cause. The toxins enter the food supply and become concentrated in certain foods. As mentioned previously when the foods are eaten, the body recognizes them as poisonous and, thus, allergic intolerance develops. Food allergies can result in dozens of respiratory symptoms. A partial list includes:

• Runny nose	• Itchy eyes
• Itchy nose	• Plugged sinuses
• Sinus infections	• Sinus headaches
• Wheezing	• Asthma attacks
• Bronchitis	• Post nasal drip
• Ear aches	• Ear discharge
• Fever/chills	• Chronic cough
• Hoarseness	• Laryngitis
• Itchy ears	• Shortness of breath
• Sore throat	• Sneezing spells
• Pneumonia	• Chest pain

From this list it becomes apparent that many lung diseases may be caused at least in part by food intolerances. Thus, it is crucial to discover the exact food intolerances in order to enhance the healing processes. Removing the food toxicities does help significantly in the cure.

The majority of food allergy tests, including the well-known scratch test, which is used by the majority of allergy specialists, are inaccurate. The scratch test is notorious for its poor accuracy for foods, with a precision of less than 30%. Rast testing is even worse, with an accuracy of only 5-10%. The fact is the results of the majority of food allergy tests may prove misleading. A specialized highly accurate food allergy test is available. Known as the Food Intolerance Test, it is a blood test requiring merely a single tube of blood. It boasts an accuracy of approximately 70% or better. The blood is processed and then carefully analyzed under a special microscope. Over 205 foods and food additives are carefully screened.

The test is based upon a principle of immunology regarding how toxins interact with the actual blood cells. Technicians view toxic reactions of food extracts against three types of blood cells: red blood cells, platelets, and white blood cells. The toxic reactions are measured as mild, moderate, and severe, and this is scored on the food chart as respectively 1, 2, or 3. A score of three indicates a severe intolerance and such foods must be avoided strictly. Ideally, all foods which score, whether 1, 2, or 3, should be avoided for at least 90 days. Afterwards, each food may be re-introduced into the diet but consumed no more than once every five days. However, if such foods cause noticeable reactions, they should be avoided indefinitely.

Currently, the Food Intolerance Test is only performed at one facility. It is a research-quality test and, therefore, is not available through standard medical laboratories. The cost is approximately $2.00 per food, which is a tremendous value considering the amount of information that is generated. Other testing may cost as much as $12.00 per food, while being less accurate. Your doctor can order this test for you by contacting:

Food Intolerance Test
1701 Golf Rd Suite 606 Tower 2
Rolling Meadows, IL 60008
(847) 640-1377

While in many individuals one test may be sufficient, it may be appropriate to repeat the test within a year. Strict avoidance of allergenic foods may result in the reversal of many of the allergies. However, there may be certain substances or foods in which the individual is allergic that should be avoided permanently, such as food additives, as is illustrated by the following case history:

Mr. J. had a history of severe sinus attacks. His sinuses would become completely plugged, causing pain and, occasionally, sinus headaches. Food intolerance testing proved he was allergic to several foods, particularly butter and cheese. Plus, he had a number of food additive allergies, including aspartame (i.e. NutraSweet). Removing the NutraSweet alone led to a significant improvement, and his sinus condition disappeared within a month.

The power of spice extracts: nature's germ killers

Spice extracts have proven germ-killing power. They don't discriminate: they kill virtually every pathogen, that is harmful germ, known. A number of spices have been studied for their germ killing powers. Chief of these is oil of wild oregano. Other extracts which kill a wide range of germs include oils of cinnamon, clove, allspice, garlic, onion, cumin, myrtle, bay leaf, sage, and thyme.

The oils from certain strains of wild oregano are potent germicides, capable of killing a wide range of germ. The use of wild oregano oil is crucial, since farm raised oregano is not as effective. As of yet no germ has been proven to resist it. However, evidence exists that an even more potent approach is to combine a number of antiseptic spices. This creates an additive, that is synergistic action, which is invaluable for the natural treatment of difficult-to-kill germs. Oregacyn is a multi-spice extract made from wild and mountain-grown spices and herbs. It offers the synergy, that is the additive action, of numerous antiseptic spices. Yet, what is of particular importance is that the spice extracts possess additional medicinal properties. They are potent antioxidants, far more powerful than mere vitamins and minerals. They are also antihistaminic, meaning they have anti-allergy properties.

Many spice extracts exert beneficial actions on the lungs, for instance, helping to thin or dry excessive mucous. Potent spice extracts, like those used in Oregacyn, also exhibit anti-pain properties. This is largely due to the incredible quantity of simple phenols they contain. This property is noticed when the pills are taken orally, usually within minutes, almost without exception. What's more, these capsules are edible, meaning that they offer health-supporting powers without the risk for serious side effects such as liver or kidney damage. The fact is with edible spice extracts there is no risk of organ damage even if large amounts are taken. Drugs destroy tissue. Spice extracts preserve it, in fact, enhance it.

Oregacyn is a special blend of multiple spices, including extracts of wild oregano (the researched P73 blend), wild sage, and mountain-grown cumin. The oils are extracted and then powdered through a proprietary process that maintains, in fact, enhances potency. Oregacyn is the most potent nutritional supplement available. Plus, it is edible, and, thus, is ideal for all ages. Use it for fast immune support, when the body needs support against stress, germs, or other immune weaknesses. It is also valuable for digestive and liver support as well as an aid to blood sugar balance. Plus, Oregacyn, being an edible multiple-spice extract, tastes great. Open the capsule and add it to soup, stir fry, cheese dip, or meat dishes. It is still useful when cooked, but, ideally, take it in the capsule as needed, one or more capsules daily. For tough situations take 2 or more capsules twice daily.

Oregacyn is not meant as a panacea. Yet, it is highly useful and is completely safe even in large amounts. Its primary use is to relieve the immune system of the burden of dealing with germs. This is because Oregacyn is germicidal, a fact which is undeniable. In contrast to drugs, which offer hundreds of side effects and may even cause death, extracts of spices are completely safe, that is they fail to cause death or organ damage. Natural spice and herbal extracts are concentrates, which offer significant antiseptic properties. Even though they are powerful health enhancers they are more ideal for internal use than the medicinal herbs. Spices are edible. So is Oregacyn.

Chapter 4

Respiratory Illnesses and Their Natural Cures

In North America respiratory conditions account for a greater number of diseases than any other category. Illnesses affecting organs such as the lungs, sinuses, ear canals, throat, etc. are the main cause of sickness. It is well known that respiratory illnesses are the number one cause of doctors' visits. Think about it. When you visit a doctor, what is it usually for? Isn't it usually for a sore throat, tonsillitis, laryngitis, flu, cold, sinus attack, ear ache, etc.? Everyone knows how much trepidation there is during cold and flu season: the hospitals and doctors' offices are often overwhelmed by the sickened. Put simply, many people fear the thought of becoming deathly ill from winter or respiratory illnesses.

Medical therapy for respiratory illnesses is lacking. Few if any cures are offered. Asthma is an excellent example. While there are numerous drugs available, as well as specialized types of respiratory therapies, the results are often poor. In fact, since the 1930s there has been a 400% rise in the death rate. The major difference is that during that era few if any pharmaceutical drugs were available.

Numerous scientific studies delineate the fact that asthma therapy increases the risks for complications as well as death. Unfortunately, the same can be said for various lung infections such as pneumonia and bronchitis. Drugs which were once highly effective are now rendered impotent, largely because of the overuse of antibiotics. Not only are the antibiotics virtually useless but the growth of certain germs may, in fact, be accelerated by them. In hospitals today resistant bacteria routinely infect the lungs and bronchial tubes, and they are impossible to kill, that is except with natural medicines. One study at Georgetown University showed that spice extracts, notably oil of wild oregano, destroyed drug resistant staph. The researchers, using a blend of wild oregano oils known as P73, were able to destroy the staph even within tissue. These incredible results illustrate the immense potential of natural compounds in the treatment of infectious disease.

There are three major categories of respiratory illnesses: the common everyday illnesses, such as colds, flu, and ear aches, which are rarely serious, the serious diseases, such as bronchitis, asthma, and pneumonia, which may be fatal, and the obscure illnesses, such as asbestosis and sarcoidois, which are frequently fatal. Cancer could be regarded as perhaps a fourth category, as there are dozens of types of respiratory cancers. What follows is a rather comprehensive list of the most common respiratory diseases and their natural, dietary, nutritional, and herbal cures.

Actinomycosis

This, as the name indicates (i.e. "mycosis"), is a type of fungus. This fungus readily grows in the respiratory system and may invade the lymph glands, especially the glands under the jaw. It is contracted as a result of exposure to grain, like grain dust. This is because the organism lives on raw grain. Thus, this disease commonly develops in farmers. It may also develop in individuals who work with flour, like workers in granaries, flour mills, or bakeries. This is because the fungus may hide on flour dust and may be inhaled.

Actinomycosis is highly invasive, although it normally only invades the tissues of individuals with weakened constitutions. It most commonly attacks the glands under the jaw and may even invade the jawbone, causing a type of osteomyelitis (bone sepsis). In many individuals this germ is an oral resident, but is not necessarily infective. Invasive dentistry may spread it, causing active infection. The teeth are a major reservoir for this germ. An infected tooth may continuously seed this organism into the bloodstream and/or tissues, causing chronic illness. The germ may also attack the tongue and throat. The lungs are readily infected, and the resulting symptoms may mimic tuberculosis. The lung infection may be difficult to eradicate, and there are no drugs for this condition. However, spice extracts destroy this fungus. Thus, the regular intake of antiseptic spice oils may prove lifesaving.

Precautions should be taken by both farmers and individuals who process/handle raw grain. If you are in this category, consider wearing a mask during potential exposure. Antifungal essential oils, like oil of lavender, oil of wild rosemary, and oil of wild oregano, should be administered. They may be taken orally or administered into the air through atomizers or vaporizers. If wearing a mask, saturate a portion of it with a few drops of oil of wild oregano (Oreganol P73). As a means of prevention take a capsule or two of Oregacyn on a daily basis. Actinomycosis is a potentially fatal disease.

Treatment protocol

Take a potent natural antiseptic, such as Oregacyn, one or more capsules twice daily. Also, use oil of wild Oreganol for oral cleansing. Add a drop or two to toothpaste or use it directly on the toothbrush. Rub a drop or two on the teeth and gums at night.

Be consistent: this is a difficult organism to eradicate. Stay on this program for at least 60 days. Also, take oil of Oreganol (P73 researched wild oregano oil blend), 4 drops under the tongue twice daily. Take also a healthy bacteria supplement, a large dose at night before bedtime. If you are exposed to grain or grain dust, take appropriate precautions like wearing a mask or maintaining proper ventilation.

Anthrax

For thousands of years anthrax has been known as a disease of animals, particularly herbivores. The anthrax bacteria, *Bacillus anthracis*, thrives in moist soil. Thus, it may contaminate grass and hay. Animals become infected by eating contaminated grass/hay or by inhaling the spores. Sheep, goats, horses, and cows are particularly susceptible to it. If the exposure is significant, anthrax infects all organs of the animals, eventually causing death.

People may occasionally contract anthrax by direct contact with animals. Those who care for animals may develop it, although it is exceptionally rare. It may be contracted from an infected animal, soil or objects that were contaminated with animal wastes, or residues in animal products, like wool or hides. The fact is during the early 1900s anthrax was known as Wool-sorter's disease. While less common, as described in the 1970s publication, *Family Health Guide*, human to human transmission may occur. This is in contrast to the current claim, which is that it is not contagious. Yet, Dr. Greer's *A Physician in the House* notes that animals which die from this disease "reek with contagion." What's more, he describes how those who handle infected tissues "are extremely liable to be poisoned...and even flies from such animals may convey (it) to human beings." Yet, admittedly today such a mode of spread would be rare.

Currently, the major concern surrounds anthrax spores. The bacteria that causes anthrax belongs to a category of germs known as spore-forming bacteria. The spore is a dormant form, meaning it may readily cause infection at a later date. According to Jordan's *General Bacteriology* the anthrax spore is one of the most resistant, that is tough-to-kill, of all bacterial forms. The typical germicides are rather impotent in destroying it. For instance, mercuric chloride, an outright poison, fails to kill it even after an hour long exposure, whereas this germicide kills virtually every other germ. However, heat and steam can kill it, although it takes a ten minute exposure to do so.

There are four forms of anthrax. The most serious is the inhalation variety, which kills most of its victims. This is caused by the direct inhalation of anthrax spores. The spores, which are sort of a bacterial seed, develop rapidly within the lungs. The lungs are thus flooded with bacteria, which suffocates the breathing mechanism. Plus, the anthrax bacteria produce potent toxins, which put the body into shock. When anthrax enters any biological fluid, as found in the lungs or blood, it reproduces in vast numbers, causing grave danger. Microbiological texts describe the observance of "enormous multiplication." They describe how the capillaries, the tiny blood vessels found in the internal organs, are "gorged"with these very large bacteria. The gastrointestinal type, which is more rare, is also highly fatal. It is usually caused by eating anthrax contaminated meat or drinking contaminated milk. Also, there is the skin type, which is characterized by the development of a circular skin lesion at the site of infection. With this type, systemic symptoms, like headache, nausea, and vomiting, may also develop. The malignant skin type may also be manifested by swelling of the tissues just below the skin, known as the subcutaneous tissues. This may result in sloughing of the skin: even gangrene.

Dr. Greer describes the transmission of cutaneous anthrax: "Wherever (it) enters the system, usually at some abraded point on the skin, a malignant pustule is formed on the fourth day after inoculation, and quickly enlarges and ulcerates and looks malignant...the nearest glands become enlarged. There is general fever and great prostration, which may be followed by collapse and death in four or five days." Interestingly, Dr. Greer described a possible cure. If the lesion was treated as soon as it developed with cautery, the progression could be halted. A common medical procedure, cautery is the use of heat directed at the skin through a hot iron or electrified probe. Perhaps this should be again investigated in the local treatment of anthrax lesions. Yet, there are less painful and more safe means of cautery: the application of phenolic extracts. Plant phenols exert a sort of "chemical cauterization" action. This action is potent and effective. While medical treatment for this condition is mandatory, the application of natural phenol-rich extracts, such as the cinnamon and oregano-based Vira Clenz and/or oil of wild Oreganol, would be an invaluable adjunct for the reversal of pustular microbial lesions.

Even if the anthrax bacteria is killed, there is another concern: the anthrax toxin. Antibiotics fail to kill it and, thus, the toxin may induce further organ damage, perhaps death. This is why it is crucial to know of the powers of natural cures. Certain herbs contain antitoxins. Turkish investigators proved that oil of wild oregano neutralized aflatoxin, one of the most potent biological toxins known. Thus, it is an ideal tonic to take in the event of exposure to a biological toxin.

Natural cures for anthrax are regarded as ineffective by the federal government. The claim is that there is a lack of proof. Yet, there is no human proof in terms of scientific studies that drugs cure it. Plus, there are no drugs capable of neutralizing anthrax toxin. Thus, their approach is to apparently keep the individual completely unaware of the possible cures in the event of a national crisis. This is a senseless approach. The fact is any agent that could be of value should be explored, that is if the objective is to protect the sanctity of human life.

The "lack of proof" statement is itself false. The fact is a number of studies have shown that anthrax may be killed with certain natural compounds, particularly spice oils. Egyptian researchers found that oils of cinnamon and cumin (both of which are found in Oregacyn) outright destroyed anthrax bacteria. Other investigators have found the bacteria's sister germ, Bacillus subtilus, is highly susceptible to oils of oregano, garlic, and thyme. The fact is natural compounds do play a significant role in protecting the body from infection. Anthrax is an infection, and it is no exception. Furthermore, in the early

1900s, when anthrax was more common in America, medical doctors used a synthetic version of the active ingredient of spice extracts, which is phenol. They gave it orally, two drops twice daily, finding it somewhat successful. According to *Beyond Antibiotics* the natural phenols of oregano are 21 times more potent that synthetic phenols. Interestingly, in the early 1900s synthetic phenol, that is carbolic acid, was relied upon for gastrointestinal anthrax. While the claim that spice extracts can cure anthrax cannot be made, further research may find that such compounds are even more potent than the synthetics. In summary, these are some of the most important issues regarding anthrax:

a) it usually presents with symptoms that in a general way mimic the flu

b) facial and nasal symptoms, such as runny nose, stuffy nose, cough, watery eyes, and sore throat probably indicate a virus, not anthrax

c) early symptoms of the inhalation variety often include deep pain in the front of the chest.

d) early signs of the skin form of anthrax are a red spot on the skin followed by a vesicle, which is usually painless and which has a center with dead cells.

e) the diagnosis requires a variety of medical tests plus a high level of suspicion. Nasal swabs only tell the degree of inhalation of spores.

Treatment protocol

The medical treatment for anthrax is the antibiotic, Cipro. Bolstering the immune system is mandatory in this disease. Take a phenolic-based multi-spice extract, such as Oregacyn, two or more capsules three times daily. In the event of dire need take two or more capsules every hour. Also, take SuperStrength Oreganol, about ten or more drops every hour. Drink also the juice of three yellow onions. You may disguise some of the taste with the juice of parsley. Also, for lung toxicity rub Respira Clenz on the chest as often as needed. Plus, take 20 drops of Respira Clenz three times daily. For skin lesions rub with SuperStrength oil of oregano and Vira Clenz as often as needed. Top with a poultice of raw honey.

Asbestos contamination (Asbestosis)

Asbestos is a fibrous compound made from minerals, mainly magnesium and silica (magnesium silicate). It is of importance, because fibers of this dangerous material easily become airborne. Inhalation of the fibers occurs mainly in factory workers. In the earlier part of the 20th century this occurred more commonly, since the dangers of asbestos fibers were largely unknown. However, today individuals who work with asbestos are carefully protected by masks and a host of strict regulations.

Usually, it takes several years of exposure to create the disease. The fibers are deposited in the bronchiole tubes. There, they stimulate scar tissue formation. The scars eventually completely consume the lungs, leading to severe breathing difficulty and, ultimately respiratory collapse and death.

Asbestos poisoning is a significant cause of death and disability. *The Chicago Tribune*, September 2001, reported the degree of human misery it can cause. An entire town, Libby, Montana, is suffering from the poisoning. Mining created dust, which residents inhaled. Some 200 people have died and thousands of others are chronically ill. This is only the tip of the iceberg. Despite extensive precautions tens of thousands of North Americans suffer from it. In the year 2000 alone work-related claims for asbestos exposure numbered 50,000. Medical costs, as well as costs for cleanup, are in the tens of billions. In Libby, Montana, the crisis is so dire that Chris Weis of the Environmental Protection Agency called it "the most severe residential exposure to a hazardous material this country has ever seen." Thus, it is no surprise that death rates from asbestosis in this town are up to 60 times greater than the national average. These people are suffering unmercifully, an agony that was largely preventable. Incredibly, up to 30% of the town members are victims of the disease. Yet, despite the fact that the risks were known, nothing was done by the government to protect the people. Only after the people themselves filed a series of lawsuits did the degree of the danger become exposed.

News reports of the lawsuits reached the EPA's Paul Peronard, who found the reports difficult to believe. Yet, when he investigated it, he found that the suffering was beyond belief. In fact, the Libby experience utterly demolished the old theories about asbestosis, that is it took prolonged regular exposure and that it took decades to develop. People became sick far more quickly than what was previously understood: in just a few years or less. Direct exposure was unnecessary. Just living in the area was enough risk. In this debacle it is expected that thousands of individuals will live in utter misery, dying a slow, writhing, miserable death, because they are suffocating to death.

To cure this condition it is necessary to dissolve the asbestos fibers. This may be accomplished by essential oil therapy. Essential oils are solvents and, thus, they help the body dissolve and decompose particulate matter. Also, they act as lymphatic stimulants: that is they aid in the flow of lymph, and it is the lymphatic ducts which become plugged in asbestosis. Thus, the regular intake of edible essential oils can prove lifesaving in this condition. The oils which are particularly valuable include oil of wild oregano as well as oils of rosemary, lavender, neroli, sage, cloves, and juniper.

Recently, an Italian study provided definitive proof of the immense value of this treatment. The study found the essential oils turn asbestos fibers into harmless polymers, which can be readily decontaminated. Unlike the fibers, the polymers are inert. Thus, they fail to induce scarring. Thus, the fatal aspects of this mineral can be neutralized precisely with natural compounds. Oil of wild oregano is the most aggressive of these depolymerizing oils.

Treatment protocol

As mentioned in ancient records wild oregano is regarded as a "cleansing" herb. Hot herbs and spices enhance blood flow, aiding in the removal of toxins. Extracts of certain spices, particularly wild oregano and thyme, offer significant solvent actions. The solvent powers of oil of wild oregano are immense. To correct this condition take edible oil of wild Oreganol, five or more drops under the tongue several times daily. For difficult cases use the SuperStrength oil of Oreganol, five drops several times daily. Take also Oregacyn, two or more capsules twice daily. Other oils which aid in the healing of lung tissue and the removal of contaminants include oils of rosemary, lavender, juniper, cloves, and sage. Respira Clenz is an essential oil combination including the edible oils of cloves, juniper, rosemary, and oregano. For additional cleansing power take 10 or more drops twice daily. Certain vitamins and minerals aid in the removal of asbestos. These include beta carotene, vitamin E, vitamin C, selenium, and zinc. Take about 25,000 I.U. of beta carotene daily along with 400 I.U. of vitamin E. Take a crude natural vitamin C supplement, such as Flavin-C, 3 capsules twice daily. Also, on a daily basis take selenium, 600 mcg and zinc, 75 mg.

Asthma

This disease is represented as sudden attacks of shortness of breath. There are numerous illnesses which may cause these attacks, but not all of them are truly asthma. For instance, a severe case of pneumonia may result in shortness of breath, as can a heart attack or congestive heart failure.

Bronchial asthma is the true type. It afflicts over ten million North Americans. The disease occurs most frequently in children and teenagers, with males being the primary victims.

It is well known that asthmatics react to things in the air. The dander of animals (i.e. animal dandruff) readily provokes it. The dander or dandruff may contain mold toxins, as well as mite toxins, and these are the likely culprits.

It has been known for decades that asthma has a major allergic component. Yet, it has also been known that infection is a major cause.

In children asthma often presents with a recurring cough for which a cause cannot be found. Yet, a recurring or persistent cough is a major symptom of disguised infection, particularly fungal or yeast infection. If the cough is not properly diagnosed and treatment offered, the infection would likely worsen, leading to intractable disease.

As early as the 1950s physicians knew that allergy to and infections by molds played an enormous role in the genesis of asthma. According to Morris Fishbein, M. D., editor of the *Medical and Health Encyclopedia,* mold sensitivity, as well as outright infection by molds/fungi, plays a "very important role." Furthermore, the editors note that a weakness in the hormonal system, or stress on this system, may either cause or precipitate asthma. The fact is a weakness in the hormonal system increases the risk for mold/fungus infection. This is largely because the hormonal system controls metabolic rate. Any weakening in the hormonal system leads to a reduction in the metabolic rate. A slow metabolism favors invasion by fungi or mold.

An old book, written in the 1930s, gives clear evidence of how atrocious the modern medical treatment is. The author notes that as a general rule physicians in the earlier part of the 20th century regarded asthma as "never fatal." The number of deaths in a year amounted to less than perhaps a few dozen. Compare this to the thousands who die yearly in the United States alone. Thus, the current medical treatment regimen for asthma is an utter failure.

Treatment protocol

Oregacyn is an invaluable supplement for asthma. Its multiple spice extracts are both antihistaminic as well as antiseptic. Plus, these extracts offer the ability to halt the production of excess mucous, while helping dislodge mucous plugs. Both Oregacyn and oil of wild Oreganol are mold killers. According to research conducted by the federal government molds are rapidly destroyed by spice extracts. Oregano oil was found to be the most potent of all. Take Oregacyn, 2 capsules twice daily. Oil of wild Oreganol is also highly effective. Take 3 or more drops under the tongue as needed. During an acute attack take it more frequently, even every few minutes. Fortunately, it is a spice and, thus, may be taken aggressively for any short term use. In reasonable amounts, like a few capsules daily, it can also be taken over a prolonged period or even indefinitely. However, even though it is only made from natural-wild spices, it is still potent. Thus, if you are taking large amounts or are taking it routinely, it is a good idea to take a natural, healthy bacteria supplement. In such circumstances take the healthy bacteria supplement, Health-Bac, right before bedtime. Research indicates that implantation of these bacteria is superior during sleep.

Raw honey may also be taken during an asthma attack. It provides energy and nutrients in an absorbable form, so direly needed to reverse this crisis. There is a contraindication: severe fungal infection, that is if the body is colonized by yeasts and fungi, which feed off of various sugars. The sugars in honey could cause a minor aggravation, although this is unusual. However, in such a case try adding a few drops of the Oreganol in the honey. This will help neutralize any sugar sensitivity.

Asthmatics usually suffer from impaired hormonal function. In particular, their adrenal glands are often weak. Thus, in order to eradicate this condition it is crucial to restore the health of these glands. The adrenal glands are weakened by stress. They are also weakened by poor diet. If a significant enough imbalance develops within these glands, they frequently become infected by parasites, bacteria, and, particularly, fungi. In addition, the adrenal glands may become infected by tuberculosis, and this is almost impossible to diagnose.

This makes sense, since asthma, being a lung disease, may be associated with a chronic low-grade TB infection. This type of TB infection is not contagious, however, it is serious enough to cause disability and/or death. However, individuals with weak adrenal glands, as represented by chronic exhaustion, weakness, depression, anxiety, and similar debilitating symptoms may have as an origin of their sickness chronic adrenal gland tuberculosis. Oregacyn is the ideal tonic for reversing this. Take it regularly for several months or until the symptoms are eliminated. The tremendous powers of Oregacyn are illustrated by the following case history:

Ms. M., a 30 year old white female, had been plagued with asthma since childhood. Mothered to death by both her mother and doctors, she was over-medicated, leading to a condition known as Cushing's Syndrome. This syndrome was due to the over-use of cortisone and Prednisone and left her blown up with water and weight. Normally a size two, she is now a size twenty. Ms. M. had constant wheezing. A friend recommended Oregacyn. Only one capsule twice daily gave her enormous relief. A colleague at work told her that after taking the Oregacyn it was the first time she noticed that she wasn't wheezing. Within five days the improvement was so dramatic that she was able to aggressively exercise at the gym without wheezing. Her mother noticed how well she was doing and broke down, crying. By consuming less than a bottle of Oregacyn, Ms. M. can safely say that her drug-resistant asthma is essentially cured.

Berylliosis

Beryllium is a metal which is usually not regarded as toxic. However, when dust from this metal is inhaled, it causes extensive lung damage. The damage is caused by scarring, which disables the ability of the lungs to supply oxygen.

The most prominent early symptom of berylliosis is severe shortness of breath, usually occurring only with exertion. Eventually, the shortness of breath is continuous. As the disease progresses the lungs fail to supply sufficient oxygen: the individual becomes cyanotic, which means the lips and fingernails become discolored (bluish). Fatigue and exhaustion become extreme. Normal activities become impossible. Memory loss may develop due to a lack of oxygen.

Treatment protocol

Edible essential spice oils are natural antiinflammatory agents, plus they possess significant solvent properties. This solvent action aids in the mobilization of the beryllium particles so they may be extracted from the lungs. Oil of wild oregano is particularly valuable, since it is a known lymph mobilizing agent. Take five or more drops of Oreganol three times daily. In a severe crisis take five or more drops every hour. Also, take the respiratory formula of spice extracts, that is Oregacyn, two capsules twice daily.

Scar tissue may be mobilized, that is dissolved. This may be accomplished through potent fruit enzymes. Papayas and pineapples produce respectively papain and bromelain, which are aggressive protein-dissolving and antiinflammatory enzymes. Scar tissue is protein, mainly collagen. Research proves that high potency papain and bromelain dissolve such tissue, even in the living body. Don't make the assumption that scar tissue is permanent. If it is provided with the appropriate tools, the body can mobilize the scar tissue. BromaZyme is a combination of high grade papain and bromelain, the highest dosage and potency available. This is a pharmaceutical-grade potency, yet it is completely natural.

Blastomycoses

This is a fungal infection that occurs mainly in regions with a moist climate. It is a serious disease and often causes fatalities. The infection attacks the lungs as well as skin. It occurs mainly in states with large river valleys, like Ohio, Iowa, Missouri, Mississippi, Kentucky, and Illinois. It is also found in the northern part of the Midwest as well as eastern Canada.

Treatment protocol

Oregacyn is the ideal treatment for this condition. Take two or more capsules twice daily. Also, take oil of wild oregano, five to ten drops twice daily. This is a serious fungal disease, and, thus, it may be necessary to take SuperStrength oil of Oreganol. For difficult cases take 10 to 20 drops of the SuperStrength twice daily.

Consume high amounts of natural vitamin C in the form of fresh orange/grapefruit juice or unsweetened currant juice (i.e. Currant-C). Eat plenty of vitamin C-rich foods such as oranges, grapefruit, kiwi fruit, broccoli, and strawberries. The reason for consuming natural instead of synthetic is that the natural is utilized more superiorly and retained in the tissues to a greater degree. What's more, it is free of side effects. Crude natural vitamin C supplements are helpful. The only ones available that contain absolutely no synthetic vitamin C are Flavin-C and Potent-C. The Flavin-C is capsules, while the Potent-C is sublingual drops. They are both unique supplements with varying benefits. Take 10 drops of Potent-C under the tongue and three capsules of Flavin-C twice daily. Selenium helps the immune system cleanse fungus: take 300 mcg of organic selenium twice daily.

Blood clots

Blood clots may originate in the lungs, or they may arise from external tissues. They may travel from these tissues and lodge in the lungs, causing potentially fatal reactions. Thus, blood clots are one of the most serious of all conditions.

This condition is thought to arise from excessive thickness or stickiness of the blood. However, trauma, which may cause internal bleeding and clotting, is an exceptionally common cause. An even more insidious cause is jet airliner flying. Flying at high altitudes causes a sort of compression of the tissues, leading to sludging. It also causes dehydration, which aggravates the dilemma. There have been a rash of cases of severe and even fatal blood clots resulting from flying. By far, this most commonly occurs from flying for prolonged periods, and mostly in those flying coach, that is in cramped quarters where there is little tendency to move about, with the middle or window seat being the most confining. People are often embarrassed or shy to make others move. However, for individuals taking prolonged flights, movement is crucial in order to prevent stagnation of blood and, therefore, blood clotting. Thus, it is mandatory on any prolonged flight to get out of the seat and move about in the aisle.

Medical treatment for clots is potent blood thinners, which may prove lifesaving. Yet, there are a wide range of natural substances with blood thinning properties. What's more, the latter are free of serious side effects. Some of these natural compounds are even capable of dissolving clots, even the deep clots found in the deepest recesses of the lungs, as is seen by the following case history:

Mr. S., a Native American of large build, developed a severely swollen calf after a thigh/pelvic injury. Incredibly, doctors diagnosed his lower leg pain as a ruptured achilles tendon. Therefore, they casted the leg, which was a dangerous thing to do. This led to further swelling. He was then correctly guided to take a high grade fruit enzyme product, pharmaceutical-grade BromaZyme, and the dosage was 4 capsules twice daily on an empty stomach. He also took the crude red grape powder (i.e. the Resvitanol), 4 capsules twice daily. Dramatically, the chronic swelling, as well as the varicose and spider veins, rapidly improved. He also noticed a 70% reduction of the problem in less than a week. He is continuing the suggested protocol and is improving daily.

Treatment protocol

Take BromaZyme biological plant enzyme complex, 3 to 4 capsules twice daily on an empty stomach. Also, take Resvitanol capsules, 3 or more capsules twice daily. Fish oils and vitamin E are anti-clotting. With fish oils, take 6 or more capsules daily and 400 I.U. of vitamin E daily. Or, for a totally natural source of the complete complement of vitamin E molecules, take

Pumpkinol (crude cold pressed pumpkinseed oil), 2 or more tablespoons daily. Eat fatty fish, like sardines, salmon, albacore tuna, herring, bluefish, etc. on a daily basis. Rub SuperStrength Oreganol on any involved area as needed. Natural vitamin C also helps prevent blood clots. This is because natural vitamin C is needed to keep the arteries from degenerating. Degenerated arteries form clots more readily, because they lose their elasticity. The loss of elasticity leads to stagnation of blood and, therefore, clot formation occurs. Take Flavin-C, three or more capsules twice daily. Also, if desired, take the crude natural and raw extract, Potent-C, ten or more drops twice daily.

Bronchitis

This term is named after a part of the lungs known as the bronchi. The bronchi are the tubes leading from the lower throat, that is the trachea, to the lung tissue. They conduct the air we breathe into the lungs so that the oxygen can be extracted by the blood. The entire system is known as the bronchial tree, in fact, schematically, it looks like an upside down tree. When the bronchi become extremely small, they lose their rigid character and instead become muscular. These tiny tubules are known as bronchioles. Bronchitis is inflammation of the bronchi and bronchioles.

Bronchitis may develop in several forms. It may be acute, meaning it suddenly develops. Usually, it is chronic, meaning it is a persistent inflammation/infection. Usually, in mild cases only the upper part of the bronchial tree is affected. However, the inflammation and/or infection may spread into the lower bronchial tree, that is the bronchioles, and this may result in serious consequences.

Often, with bronchitis breathing is terribly restricted. It is the inflammation, soreness, and cough that are particularly distressing. The cough may be highly distressing and racking; there is often pain and a sensation of rawness behind the breastbone. Fever is rare, but the individual may become fatigued easily.

The pattern of the cough is typical. At first there is little or no sputum, but the cough is painful. Eventually, the cough becomes productive, and frothy whitish sputum is produced. Later, the color changes, and it may become yellow or more rarely green. When this happens, the pain of the cough is reduced. These symptoms are classic for acute or chronic bronchitis. There is a difference between this presentation and that of pneumonia. Usually, similar symptoms occur with pneumonia, but fever, chills, and sweating also develop.

Treatment protocol

Multiple spice extracts have been proven by scientific studies to kill a wide range of germs. A federal government study proved that both molds and bacteria, major causes of bronchial conditions, were killed. Take Oregacyn, 2 capsules twice daily, and increase the dosage if necessary. Take also oil of wild oregano, five drops twice daily. Raw honey may be helpful to ease symptoms. A rich tasting wild oregano honey is available and can only be ordered via the mail. To order call 1-800-243-5242.

Bronchiectasis

This is a disease of the bronchial tubes. It is signified by the enlargement or weakening of certain bronchial tubes, which balloon out, forming cavities. These cavities may be seen on x-ray. This is a problem, because the bronchial tubes are normally elastic, that is tight-walled. In fact, their circumscribed size enables them to maintain proper function. This allows them to remain relatively free of debris, that is the cilia along with the muscular contractions propel debris back out of the lungs. However, when they balloon out, debris, secretions, and, thus, germs accumulate. The accumulated material festers, causing bad breath. Foul smelling sputum may be produced.

In the 1940s it was discovered that sinus infections may induce bronchiectasis. The germs from the infected sinuses seed the bronchial tubes, causing widespread damage. The germs apparently destroy the muscular tissues of the bronchial tubes, leading to bronchiectasis. The responsible germs are now known: fungi. This makes sense, because fungi are notorious for their ability to produce proteolytic enzymes. These enzymes are capable of digesting living proteins, including the smooth muscle which lines the bronchioles. Once this muscle is lost, there is no means for the bronchial tubes to retain their strength or shape and, therefore, they degenerate.

The original site of these fungal infections may be the teeth, from which the organisms seep into the sinuses. Invasive dentistry may rapidly spread the infections, leading to acute or chronic lung or sinus infections. If the sinus infection remains chronic and untreated, bronchiectasis may eventually develop.

Treatment protocol

Oregacyn is the ideal oral therapy for this condition: take one or more capsules twice daily. Also, take oil of wild oregano, three to five drops under the tongue twice daily. For more difficult conditions take five to ten drops twice daily. Also, take a natural-source vitamin C supplement, like Flavin-C, six or more capsules daily. Vitamin C is needed to maintain the strength of the bronchial tubes. Vitamin A is needed for healthy bronchioles. If you have chronic lung disease and/or bronchiectasis, take 5,000 to 10,000 I.U. daily. Or, instead of the supplement, eat organic liver, six to eight ounces twice weekly. Also, take a crude natural beta carotene supplement, 25,000 I.U. daily.

Cancer of the lungs

This is one of the greatest and most severe of all modern epidemics. Particularly common in smokers, it is also common in those exposed to second hand smoke as well as industrial workers who are exposed to noxious fumes.

There are two major types of lung cancer: the type that originates directly within the lungs and the metastatic type, that is the type that is seeded to the lungs. Regarding the latter the cancer starts in outside organs, like in the prostate, breast, or bone, and is carried to the lungs via the blood or lymph.

Lung metastases develop in millions of Americans yearly. However, these cancers may not provoke symptoms and, thus, are occasionally discovered on routine X-rays.

Primary cancers usually develop within the bronchial tubes. From here they invade the lymphatics, which disseminate the cancer throughout the lungs. The lymph glands near the tumor become infiltrated by these cells. Shortness of breath may develop, which is caused by the swelling of the lymph glands and from the mechanical blockage of the tumor in the bronchial tubes. Unless this tumor is aggressively treated, it may eat through the bronchial tubes and consume the lung tissue, making it virtually impossible to breathe.

Cancer of the lungs is usually regarded as routinely fatal. In medicine it is believed that nothing can be done about it. Yet, physicians are unaware of the immense power of natural cures. Nature offers a wide range of cancer answers. Thus, there is no need to lose hope. In fact, cancer is merely a disease, no more threatening than any other. If the proper treatment is applied, a cure can be achieved and in many instances rather rapidly. Native Americans cured thousands of cases of cancer long before modern medicine. Their therapies included incantations, positive thinking, and medicinal herbs.

Oil of wild oregano, as well as the multiple spice extract, Oregacyn, is potent natural tonic for the lung tissues. To greatly boost the health of the lungs and cleanse them of dangerous toxins take large amounts of these tonics. The Juice of Oregano is also an invaluable tonic. Studies in Turkey indicated that it is a powerful anti-cancer agent.

Treatment protocol

Stress must be minimized or preferably eliminated: it is the primary cause of cancer. If you are a worrier, defeat this habit. A good book for this purpose is Dale Carnegie's *How to Stop Worrying and Start Living*. If you smoke, stop immediately. If those close to you smoke, they should be prohibited from doing so. If they cannot stop their habit, make them smoke outdoors at a distance from the house. Cigarette smoke is exceptionally toxic and is the primary chemical cause of lung cancer. Juice of Oregano has significant anecdotal history as a cancer remedy. As of yet, however, there is no government approval for such a treatment. Even so, it may be considered an immune tonic. Drink 2 to 6 ounces twice daily. Also, drink Juice of Rosemary,

4 ounces daily. Rosemary has been shown to be one of nature's most potent anti-cancer agents. Take also the multiple spice extract, that is Oregacyn, 3 capsules twice daily. Increase the intake of dark green leafy vegetables and vitamin C-rich fruit, particularly organic kiwi, papaya, grapefruit, blueberries, and strawberries. Eat a large organic spinach salad daily topped with extra virgin olive oil and vinegar.

Take precautions to protect yourself against second hand smoke. Do not consume nitrated or smoked meats: they are primary cancer promoters. Eliminate the intake of all refined vegetable oils and hydrogenated oils. Butter, tallow, and extra virgin olive oil are allowed. Furthermore, regarding spice extracts take as much as is needed to improve overall health. The oregano oil may be taken profusely, like a few drops every hour.

Candida

Candida is a yeast, which infects human tissues. It is an enormous cause of human disease and disability as well as death. Candida is one of the most common pathogens of the lungs. It may infect virtually any organ, including the blood, spleen, intestines, esophagus, stomach, bladder, kidneys, and even the brain.

Candida has been implicated in a number of respiratory diseases, particularly asthma, sinusitis, ear infections, and bronchitis. It may also cause a type of pneumonia, which is usually fatal. While with the standard medical therapy it is difficult to kill, research proves that spice extracts are highly effective against it. Preliminary research indicates that such extracts are just as effective as the standard drugs.

The components of Oregacyn kill Candida. The fact that spice oil extracts kill Candida was proven by Georgetown University.

The extracts were so effective that they were shown in preliminary research to completely clear yeasts from organs and tissues, while improving the health of the test animals.

Treatment protocol

Take a multiple spice extract, that is Oregacyn, two capsules twice daily. Also, take oil of wild Oreganol, five to ten drops under the tongue twice daily. For difficult cases use the SuperStrength oil of oregano, five or more drops under the tongue twice daily.

Colds

No one knows for sure what causes the common cold. What is known is that it is an infectious disease, probably a virus. However, recent evidence points to the role of fungi and fungal toxins in causing cold, as well as flu, symptoms.

Theories for the cause of colds goes back thousands of years. A book written in the early 1900s, *How to Get Well*, by Dr. W. A. Evans, offers some insight into past and, seemingly viable, theories. Here is what Emeritus Eliot said in the early 1900s:

> "People who live in the forest, in open barns, or with open windows do not catch cold...(colds are)...caused by impure air, lack of exercise, or overeating." The Naturalist John Muir observed, "as long as I camp out in the mountains without tents or blankets, I get along very well, but the very minute I get into a house and have a warm bed and begin to live on fine food, I get into a draft and the first thing I know

I am coughing and sneezing and threatened with (infection). Also at the turn of the century Irving Foster noted that people who live outdoors are virtually immune from colds. A chart is listed showing the incidence of colds/flu. Their findings were as follows: impure air causes respiratory diseases. They failed to determine the culprit, but they did discern much of the cause. Pneumonia and bronchitis were found to occur mainly in the winter, when people "house themselves up and breathe the foul air of unventilated rooms."

What is known is that the common cold is highly contagious. People who are indoors during winter months are the most vulnerable, since this wintry infection is readily spread by close contact, especially through coughing or sneezing.

Cold victims suffer miserably, although it is a rather limited disease. It strikes the head and neck, and the nasal passages are severely affected.

That weather changes are involved in the creation of colds has been suspected since the time of Hippocrates. Most colds occur towards the middle of fall, for instance, in October. The incidence rises again in January and February, climaxing in March. During the spring and summer the incidence is low. From this it is easy to understand the role of the sun. When there is plenty of sunlight, the incidence of colds plummets. Thus, cold weather itself is not the cause of colds. People who are constantly outdoors during the winter rarely get colds. For instance, in their native environment the Inuit (formerly known as Eskimos) have always been cold free. When they were originally visited by Western explorers, they caught colds from them.

This shows that colds are transmissible, but it also proves that cold weather or dry cold air by itself fails to cause colds. There must be other factors. For instance, while colds do develop when the weather turns cold, this is also when people spend a greater amount of time indoors. It is also when they first turn on their furnaces after months of inactivity. Most furnaces are in basements, which are excellent repositories of dust and, particularly, mold. The fact is mold counts in houses may reach astronomically high levels as the result of forced air heat, especially if the filters are poorly cleaned and/or if the furnace is in a basement with high mold counts. When the molds are inhaled, they attach to the lung and bronchial tissues. There, they reproduce, secreting poisons. The poisons debilitate the immune system, increasing the vulnerability to infections by cold viruses and other pathogens.

One noted British researcher, Dr. A. V. Hill, believes that cold weather instigates colds, because people are primarily indoors. They stay for longer periods in warm and stuffy rooms, failing to ventilate them. They perspire, giving off noxious gases. They sneeze and cough, liberating pathogens, which, if not ventilated, multiply indoors.

During cold weather they rely on forced heat furnaces and, habitually, fail to open windows. This was confirmed by Dr. E. O. Jordan of the University of Chicago, who found that 90% of colds occur when there is minimal or no ventilation and when windows are never opened, like during the chilly part of the fall as well as the winter. This is particularly true in office buildings, where it is socially unacceptable to open windows on blustery, cold days. This is proof that a change in weather, that is a change in human habits based upon the weather, is a definite factor in causing colds. The fact is people who live and work in crowded surroundings are the primary cold victims.

Poor hygiene increases the risks for developing colds. The hands are constantly covered with the residues from, for instance, a sneeze or from touching the nasal region, mouth, etc. Then, the contaminated hand induces transmission through contact with other individuals through hugs, pats, handshakes, kisses, etc. or through touching inanimate objects, like railings or doorknobs. The cold germs remain viable for at least a few hours and are readily transmitted to other individuals.

Crowding is a major cause of colds, but this is only because crowding increases the ease for their spread. Germs are spread mainly through the air, arising from the breath of various humans or through sneezing or coughing. However, crowded places may also place people at risk, because of contaminated inanimate objects, including doorknobs and toilet seats.

Germs are invasive. Their objective is to attack and colonize. They lie in wait for a vulnerable subject. If you live or work in a crowded environment, place great importance upon proper hygiene. This will help minimize the potential for exposure. Yet, even the most fastidious individual may fall victim to the germs found in a crowded environment. This is because most infectious diseases are airborne, and, thus, the infections may develop in spite of all precautions. This is why hygienic individuals may readily develop infections after riding on a subway or bus or flying in an airplane. In other words, the individual may be fastidious in his/her hygiene and still become infected simply because the air is foul. However, there is a simple solution: antiseptic protection.

Cold weather and/or being outdoors in the winter, that is

being exposed to cold air is not the main cause of colds. In fact, spending time outdoors is preventive. This is because fresh air cleans the sinuses, lungs, and remainder of the respiratory tract. In contrast, indoor air spreads colds, especially in the fall and winter. As stated previously one problem is that during cold weather furnaces are used. In causing sinus or cold/flu symptoms forced heat furnaces are one of the greatest villains. The dry heat desiccates the mucous membranes, weakening them. Mucous membranes must be moist to provide the proper anti-viral defenses. This may be corrected by adding moisture to the air, enough to prevent drying of the membranes but not too much, which could encourage the growth of molds.

The lack of sunlight during fall/winter predisposes to colds. Germs are neutralized by sunlight. Even though there is sunlight during this time the power of the rays is significantly diminished, because of the increased distance of the sun from the earth. In other words, when sunlight is diminished germs flourish, not so much outdoors but indoors. During the cold winter period the outdoor air is relatively sterile. However, the combination of the warmth from artificial heating plus a lack of sunlight allows germs to multiply indoors in vast numbers. There is another reason that a lack of sunlight increases the risks: a reduction in metabolism. Sunlight is needed to boost the metabolic rate. When this rate slows, the immune system is more sluggish, and blood flow is reduced. When blood flow is impaired, there is less oxygen delivered to the tissues. Oxygen is one of nature's most powerful antiseptics.

For modern medicine the treatment of colds has always been a conundrum. Vaccines have been attempted, but these have proven mostly useless. These vaccines have been made using specific cold viruses. Their failure is in part due to the fact that colds are caused by a number of organisms, and not just viruses.

Molds are a major cause of colds and cold-like symptoms. The molds are highly toxic to the immune system. They suppress immunity, making the body more vulnerable to viral attack. If the molds are killed, that is cleansed out of the body, the cold virus cannot attack you.

As early as the 1940s medical doctors recommended colon cleansing as a treatment for colds. The idea is that toxins in the colon depress the immune system, increasing the risks for infection. Enemas and laxatives were administered. These seem to have a positive effect. Yet, it is reasonable to presume that occasionally cleansing the colon through herbal laxatives or enemas may aid in prevention. In the 1940s and 50s prodigious amounts of lemonade and orange juice were recommended with definite results. The benefit is largely due to the content of immune boosting vitamins, like folic acid and vitamin C. If using lemonade, do not add sugar. Make your own lemonade from real lemons. Sweeten with raw honey or stevia. Sugar depresses immunity, prolonging the illness. The use of hot spices on the feet is a valuable and time-honored aid. I found this recommendation in a medical book written in the 1940s. The doctors recommended bathing the feet in mustard baths. Even superior to this is the use of oil of wild oregano. In a foot soak add about 50 drops. Soak for an hour or two. Results will be noticed fairly quickly, like within two hours.

As mentioned previously a lack of fresh air is an enormous cause of disease but, today, this is rarely recognized. People stay much of their lives indoors in poorly ventilated facilities. Some office buildings offer no access to outside air. This extreme lack of ventilation increases the risks for a variety of illnesses, including asthma, colds, flu, sinus problems, migraine headaches, bronchitis, pneumonia, and even tuberculosis.

In the past it was clearly known that stagnant, contaminated, and/or polluted air causes ill health. A book written in 1884, Smith's *Human Body and its Health*, describes how this occurs. In a section called Waste Matters Given Off By the Lungs a number of facts are provided. The lungs are described as a gas-exchanging organ, which siphons in oxygen and expels carbon dioxide and other useless gases. In fact, the lungs play a major role in aggressively expelling waste material. Water is also expelled with each exhalation and usually this water is permeated with noxious gases.

Incredibly, within 24 hours the average human expels through the lungs up to a pint of wastewater. When we breath, we take in a combination of mainly oxygen and nitrogen. When we exhale, the air has lost oxygen and gained carbon dioxide plus water vapor as well as various noxious and potentially toxic gases, like methane and pentane. What's more, according to Smith, who was a human hygiene expert, expelled air is "not fit to be breathed again...(and it is so useless)...we could not live in it...moreover, it is injurious."

The accumulation of large amounts of this human effluent can be catastrophic. Smith describes a case in Calcutta: nearly 150 men were packed into a room only 18 x18 feet, that is the size of a large bedroom. Within 24 hours, some 120 men died. Even in 1884 Smith regarded fresh air as a rare commodity, stating that virtually everyone living in the modern world suffers constantly from a lack of it and that its importance should always be kept in mind. Vague symptoms, he says, are likely due to a lack of fresh air, symptoms such as a general sensation of illness, mental fatigue, drowsiness, and lack of desire to exercise. A few deep breaths of the fresh air outdoors could quickly regenerate the health and eliminate the symptoms.

Treatment protocol

Extracts of wild and mountain-harvested spices are potential cures for the common cold. In fact, colds are no contest for the nasal and sinus cleansing powers of Oregacyn as well as the Oreganol oil. Indeed, the positive experiences of hundreds of thousands of individuals prove that oil of Oreganol, and similar spice extracts, cure the common cold. The fact is the antiviral and cold virus destroying actions of this oil are indisputable. What's more, crude spice extracts are a type of general germicide, capable of destroying cold viruses and flu viruses as well as molds. Thus, all the various causes of cold/flu syndrome are destroyed.

Oregano, cinnamon, cloves, and sage are potent antihistaminic substances, plus they contain compounds, notably terpenes, long chain alcohols, flavonoids, and phenolic agents, which boost the body's anti-viral defenses. Oregacyn, rich in antiseptic spices, including sage, cinnamon, and oregano, is a fast acting means to obliterate both cold symptoms and the germs which instigate it. Take 1 or 2 capsules three times daily. Also, oil of wild oregano is useful. For best results take the oil frequently, like every few hours. Also, rub the oil on the feet morning and night. Foot rubs with hot spices have been used in the treatment of colds for hundreds of years.

Raw honey is an excellent medicine for respiratory conditions particularly colds. According to Loran in *Health Through Rational Diet* honey's content of antibiotic acids, particularly formic acid, accounts for much of its antiseptic qualities. Plus, formic acid is apparently an antidote to excessive mucous and is very soothing for clearing the throat and sinuses. Honey is certainly a sugar, but it is the most natural type available. It is readily digested and causes less stress upon the body than refined sugar. Honey is gathered as nectar from flowers. The flowers contain various nutritive and antibiotic substances, which the bees concentrate. The formic acid is synthesized by the bees, which secrete it into the honey.

The antiseptic and medicinal properties of honey are largely dependent upon the type of plants visited by the bees. A wild oregano honey is available. Made from oregano and other antiseptic plants, this honey is exceptionally rich in organic acids, such as formic acid, as well as minerals. It is a dark colored honey, indicating the intensity of its mineral content. Wild oregano honey must be ordered via mail order: 1-800-243-5242.

Hot lemonade may also be a useful tonic. Do not add sugar; either drink it straight or add raw honey. To make this, thoroughly squeeze the juice of four lemons and add to a quart of water. Also, add a pinch of sea salt. Sweeten with honey to desired sweetness and drink a quart daily.

Be sure to fast from solid food. During colds eating dense foods, like meat, cheese, butter, eggs, as well as rich sauces, will aggravate them.

Collapsed lung

This serious condition is becoming increasingly common. It is usually caused by trauma. However, infection may also cause it.

The lungs are highly resistant to collapse. This is because they are a tough elastic organ. They have a natural tendency to stay inflated. This is because the lungs are surrounded by a vacuum, which keeps them inflated. However, if this vacuum is compromised, the lungs may collapse. This usually occurs from direct trauma. However, certain lung diseases, as well as sudden infections, may damage the outer lung layers, and a hole may be formed, breaking the vacuum.

A type of collapsed lung may occur in tuberculosis. It happens without warning. It is caused by the ulceration of the outer layers of the lung, which destroys the natural vacuum. This usually occurs in people over 45.

Another type develops in younger people, including athletes. It also occurs without warning. Healthy college students are the usual victims. It begins with a sudden episode of chest pain, difficulty breathing, and, eventually, cyanosis. A smoldering unknown lung infection may have precipitated it, although excessive alcohol intake and/or binge drinking may be the primary precipitant.

Treatment protocol

Vitamin C may prevent the breakdown of the outer lung layers. It is also needed to maintain the integrity of the lung's elastic components. A lack of vitamin C leads to the breakdown of lung tissues. Take a crude natural vitamin C, such as Flavin-C, three capsules twice daily. Rosemary is an invaluable lung tonic. Take oil of wild rosemary, 10 drops twice daily under the tongue.

Also, drink Juice of Rosemary, two ounces twice daily. To cleanse the lungs of infection take Oregacyn, two or more capsules three times daily. Take also Respira Clenz, a potent essential oil combination, ten or more drops twice daily. Fatty acids, such as lecithin and essential fatty acids, may help re-inflate the lungs by providing those slippery substances known as surfactants. Take lecithin, 3 heaping tablespoons daily. As a source of crude essential fatty acids as well as vitamin E take Pumpkinol (crude mountainous pumpkinseed oil), three tablespoons daily. Also, take fish oils, 6 to 10 capsules daily. Oregacyn may also prove helpful: take 1 or 2 capsules twice daily.

Cough

A cough is merely a symptom. It may be generated by a vast number of illnesses or conditions. Cough can be an extremely serious symptom, signaling potentially fatal disease of the lungs. Or, it may be caused by something completely innocuous such as excessive wax build-up in the ears.

Usually, suppressing a cough, that is with potent sedative medications, is a bad idea. The cough may be a good sign, that is that the body is attempting to rid itself of a toxin, germ, or irritant. If the noxious agent is eradicated, the cough disappears. Thus, the cause of the cough should be resolved and/or the irritant should be cleansed. Though wild oregano may eliminate a cough, it does so by eradicating the most common cause: germs.

Treatment protocol

Chronic cough is a signal that something is irritating the lungs, usually an allergen, toxic chemical, or microbe. Oregacyn is a natural antioxidant, anti-allergen, anti-toxin, and anti-microbial. To eradicate the cause of the cough take 2 capsules twice daily. For severe unrelenting cough take higher amounts, like 2 or 3 capsules three times daily.

Raw honey, especially antiseptic honeys, like wild thistle and oregano honeys, may be helpful. Certainly, the raw honey will help soothe the throat and is ideal for irritated throat due to repeated coughing. Take the honey direct, like a teaspoon melted into the mouth or in warm herbal tea. Or, it may be stirred into warm salt water or vinegar water.

Cystic fibrosis

This is a hereditary disease of certain glands in the body known as exocrine glands, that is the glands that secrete digestive juices, mucus, tears, etc. The main gland affected is the pancreas, however, the function of the lungs is also severely compromised. This is because in cystic fibrosis there is a defect in mucous secretion. The mucous is extremely sticky and thick, which causes a wide range of disabilities. This thick mucus plugs the various ducts, leading to swelling, scarring, and permanent damage. The organs become so damaged that they fail to produce their secretions. For instance, the pancreas fails to produce enzymes, and the lungs fail to produce sufficient quantities of protective mucous. The thick mucous which is produced is abnormal in chemistry. It fails to protect the lungs from germs, plus it plugs various lung tubules, allowing germs to multiply. The lack of enzymes impairs digestion, leading to malnutrition and outright vitamin deficiency.

The digestion of fat is particularly impaired, which leads to a deficiency of fat soluble vitamins, notably vitamins A, E, and D. The lack of vitamin A is of particular concern, since this vitamin is required for the creation of healthy lung cells and for protecting the lungs against infection.

In cystic fibrosis virtually all of the organs are negatively affected. The greatest disruption occurs in the exocrine glands. "Exo" means exterior. Thus, the exocrine glands are the ones which secrete their productions outward. For instance, the pancreas produces enzymes, which it secretes into the intestines. This organ's function is greatly impaired in cystic fibrosis. Other glands which produce outgoing secretions include the sweat glands, mucous glands, breasts, and salivary glands. All of these glands fail to produce sufficient quantities of their excretions, plus they tend to degenerate, becoming scarred or plugged. This plugging, which occurs in the ducts of these various glands, is the key feature of this disease. Clogged ducts breed germs. Thus, infections are the major cause of illness and death. This illustrates that the key to aiding these individuals is to keep the secretions flowing and prevent scar formation.

The sweat glands are also negatively affected. These glands lose their ability to reabsorb salt. Thus, salt is easily lost and salt deficiency, that is a deficiency of sodium and chloride, is common. The lack of sodium and chloride greatly disturbs body function. Thus, the regular intake of large amounts of salt helps prevent a variety of complications.

Aggressive care is necessary for individuals to remain as healthy as possible. In the past the death rate was exceedingly high, with victims usually dying by early adulthood. However, today with proper care sufferers can live a relatively normal life. Nutritional and herbal remedies have had an enormously positive impact upon the course of this disease. Without proper supplementation and dietary measures cystic fibrosis patients rapidly degenerate. Mechanical aids, such as breathing exercises, massage, and respiratory therapies, are also useful, since they assist greatly in keeping the secretions flowing and preventing mucous plugs. It may also be helpful to naturally bolster thyroid function. This is because this gland controls both excretory actions as well as the quality and consistency of body secretions.

Treatment protocol

Oil of wild Oreganol is absolutely essential for this condition and may often prove lifesaving. Oregacyn is also particularly valuable, as it helps cleanse the body of deep-seated pathogens. Use also the oil as a foot massage; there are hundreds of lung reflexes there. Rub preferably the SuperStrength oil of Oreganol on the feet once or twice daily. After rubbing it on the feet in the morning, put on stockings. This will hold the oil on the region, offering a sort of daylong therapy.

Vitamin-mineral therapy is essential, as is the intake of fatty acids. Fat soluble vitamins and fatty acids must be taken in a mycelized form. Also, a mycelized form of wild oregano oil is now available (for more information call 1-800-243-5242, as it is not in stores yet).

Salt depletion is common and dangerous. Sea salt should be routinely added to food. A high quality kelp supplement, such as ThyroKelp, should be taken on a daily basis (2 to 12 capsules daily). For infants or small children such capsules may be opened and added to food. Kelp is a rich source of iodine, sodium, and chloride, which are direly needed by cystic fibrosis patients. Commercial kelp is often contaminated with high levels of arsenic. The kelp in Thyrokelp has been assayed and shown to be free of such industrial contaminants.

A high protein diet has been found to be the most beneficial for this condition. Refined carbohydrates, such as white flour, rice, and sugar, must be strictly avoided. The fact is grains are the most difficult of all foods to digest and, thus, should be restricted or avoided completely. Corn and beans should also be avoided. This is because these foods commonly cause allergic intolerance, plus they are high in substances called lectins. The lectins cause irritation of the mucous membranes. The ideal diet is rich in fresh fish, red meat, poultry, fresh vegetables, and fresh fruit. Milk products that may be tolerated include yogurt and goat's milk. Eggs may also be tolerated. Although milk and eggs, are nutritionally rich, an allergic reaction to these foods is common and, thus, they may need to be avoided. If milk is strictly restricted, be sure to provide a calcium supplement as well as supplemental vitamin D.

The diet should be free of foods which clog intestinal function, that is foods which are difficult to digest. Grains are among the most difficult of all foods to digest. As mentioned previously, this is partly because grains contain lectins, which are sticky substances that become like glue within the intestines.

Many individuals have extreme difficulty digesting grains. Celiac disease is a specific syndrome in which the ingestion of grains destroys the intestinal lining. In this syndrome individuals have toxic reactions to any grains which contain the protein known as gluten. This is one of the few diseases that is much like cystic fibrosis in its presentation.

Ideally, for cystic fibrosis patients all gluten containing grains, that is wheat, oats, rye, kamut, spelt, and barley, should be strictly avoided. Interestingly, the aforementioned grains are also high in lectins. Corn and beans, which are also high in lectins (but contain no gluten), should also be avoided.

Emphysema

This is one of the most devastating of all lung diseases. It is manifested by total destruction of lung cells, that is the alveoli.

The lung is an elastic organ. Under a microscope tiny air organs are revealed, which expand and contract with every breath. These are known as the air vesicles or alveoli. It is a beautiful sight to watch these microscopic organs expand and contract with every inhalation and exhalation.

The alveoli are highly vulnerable to toxic insults. In particular cigarette smoke destroys them. If enough of the alveoli are destroyed, emphysema develops. Thus, emphysema is defined as the loss of the normal elastic cells of the lungs. When these cells are destroyed, the lung enlarges, pushing the ribs out. That is why emphysema patients are barrel chested.

It is a little known fact that germs can cause or accelerate emphysema. Mold is one of the most insidious toxins that can can cause it. Certain molds are highly invasive, that is they aggressively attack and destroy tissue. They may, in fact, feed off of human cells, including the nutrient-rich lung cells. Molds secrete enzymes, which digest, that is destroy, human tissue.

With emphysema victims there is yet another dilemma: oxidative damage to the lungs. This may be evidence that the body and specifically lung tissue is deficient in critical antioxidants such as selenium, glutathione, vitamin C, and vitamin E. Antioxidants limit and, in some instances, reverse the oxidative damage occurring in the lungs from various insults such as infection, polluted air, and cigarette smoke.

While the vitamins and minerals are fairly potent antioxidants, natural plant chemicals may be regarded as superpotent. Numerous natural plant chemicals, such as phenols and flavonoids, have been shown to be up to 100 times more effective than vitamins or minerals. The ideal approach is to take a combination of antioxidant vitamins, minerals, and plant compounds in order to protect the lung tissue to the utmost.

Due to the destruction of the elastic walls of the lungs, as well as the alveoli, the ability of the lungs to expand and contract is severely impaired. Thus, the inability to expel inhaled air is one of the cardinal symptoms of emphysema. In essence once the air is inhaled, it becomes trapped within the lungs. Individuals with emphysema complain of shortness of breath and a feeling of suffocation. This trapping of air and suffocation makes emphysema one of the most gruesome of all diseases known.

Cigarette smoking is the primary cause of this condition. This type of smoke is so profoundly toxic to the lungs that it causes massive inflammation, leading to scarring and cellular breakdown. Immediately after inhaling it—even the amount from a single puff—cell death begins. Plus, cigarette smoke destroys vitamins C and E, needed to keep the alveoli in top condition. A single cigarette destroys as much as 30 mg of vitamin C and 3 mg of vitamin E. When these vitamins are depleted, these delicate air sacs degenerate, and, thus, they cannot properly deliver oxygen. The loss of these air sacs leads to disruption in the function of the entire body, since the body's ability to deliver oxygen to the blood is lost. If you smoke, quit. Otherwise, you risk permanent and irreversible lung damage and, certainly, premature death.

Treatment protocol

Take the antioxidant and antiseptic tonic, Oregacyn, 2 or more capsules twice daily. Also, rub oil of Oreganol and/or oil of rosemary on the chest at night. You may choose to add these oils into a heavy fat, like coconut fat or cocoa butter and rub onto the chest. Use the researched/tested Oreganol oil of oregano, which is 100% wild. Greek research determined that wild oregano may be up to 400% more powerful than the commercial type. The latter is often farm-raised, and the chemistry of farm raised is considerably different than that of the wild type. This certainly explains the difference in efficacy. The oil of oregano may also be taken internally, for instance, 3 to 5 drops twice daily under the tongue. Usually, the oil helps improve breathing dramatically. Avoid exposure to noxious fumes, especially cigarette smoke. Also, take selenium, 400 mcg daily and natural vitamin C (such as Potent-C drops or Flavin-C capsules), about 200 mg of natural vitamin C daily. If taking the Potent-C, the dose is 3 to 4 teaspoons daily and with Flavin-C, about 8 capsules daily. In order to speed healing or regeneration, even large amounts may be necessary. Flavin-C and Potent-C are completely non-toxic and are well tolerated by individuals with sensitive systems. In addition, take natural-source vitamin E, 400 to 800 I.U. daily as well as natural-source beta carotene, 50,000 I.U. daily. BromaZyme, a potent natural source of fruit enzymes, may aid in the dissolution of scar tissue as well as in the liberation from the lungs of toxins, particularly tar and particulate matter: take 3 capsules twice daily on an empty stomach.

Demolition lung (World Trade Center Syndrome)

It has been long known that workers in the demolition field suffer a specific respiratory syndrome. This is due to the inhalation of the dust liberated from construction and demolition.

A similar syndrome has resulted from the World Trade Center disaster. This debacle resulted in the liberation of vast quantities of airborne particles, many of them poisonous. Asbestos, silica, lead, cadmium, volatile hydrocarbons, petrochemical fumes: all were liberated. Obviously, the people in the inner city inhaled these substances in relatively large quantities. The plumes of dust and fumes floated throughout the city, contaminating the lungs of hundreds of thousands of people. The result may be thousands of cases of chronic lung disease: a dangerous and insidious epidemic.

According to the *Chicago Tribune* workers as well as residents near the sight are becoming increasingly ill. The dust and toxins released by the collapsing towers have made them ill, creating fears of long-term diseases such as emphysema, asthma, and lung cancer. Anyone who worked on the site and failed to use a respirator is at a high risk for inhalation illness including asbestosis, silicosis, and lung infection.

Asbestos is particularly dangerous. However, the dust of vaporized concrete is equally vile. Imagine what this must do to to the lungs. Finely milled concrete flour in the air is inhaled into the moist lungs. The concrete dust, rich in silica and other damaging minerals, mixed with the moisture within the lungs congeals into a concrete-like compound, causing massive lung irritation and leading to swelling, inflammation, and scarring. The Trade Center site is asbestos contaminated. In fact, contamination in lower Manhattan is rife. The authorities cannot be relied on in their lackadaisical attitude. It is obviously contaminated. The 1970s era building made extensive use of asbestos in pipe insulation and for other purposes. The vaporization of any such massive site must lead to serious pollution, since today's high-rise buildings contain billions of pounds of hazardous materials. Government firms may have seemingly minimal concern for the level of contamination. In contrast, reputable private firms have discovered that the levels are exceptionally high, as would be expected from the types and age of the involved buildings. Informing the public of the level of poison is helpful, not harmful

Certain agencies have reported that air in lower Manhattan is safe. Yet, thousands of New York City residents are reporting lung symptoms, all of which have developed since the collapse. In fact, it is less stressful to admit the existence of a problem, even if there is little the government can do about it. For instance, local doctors in inner Manhattan are convinced that the air is poisonous. Dr. Stephen Levin, medical director of occupational and environment diseases at Mount Sinai Medical Center, claims that the air is causing serious respiratory ailments. The fact is nearly half of all rescue workers, some 5,000 individuals, developed chronic lung symptoms as a result of persistently inhaling the toxic and dust-contaminated air. This degree of contamination is causing a significant syndrome, which will likely plague thousands of individuals for years, perhaps lifetimes. This illustrates the importance of utilizing natural healing aids to assist the ability of the lungs to heal. What's more, according to the WB11 News, thousands of New York City firemen and women are suffering from a constellation of respiratory symptoms, which, because of their timing and unusual nature, have been coined The World Trade Center Syndrome.

There is great benefit in evaluating these issues in a non-emotional and unbiased manner. Long term damage is likely, and a thorough understanding of the causes of this syndrome could help prevent disability as well as premature death. As a result of a factual representation of these issues, ultimately, much agony, as well as many lives, will be saved. Any attempt to repress information could be devastating. This is because the appropriate action must be taken to reverse the forthcoming health crises. In fact, without effective or curative treatment, potentially hundreds of thousands of New York City residents could develop chronic debilitating lung diseases.

Even with the degree of poisoning experienced by New York City residents permanent pain and agony is unnecessary. This is because certain natural compounds speed the healing of lung tissue and aid in the removal of noxious compounds.

Treatment protocol

Massive doses of certain natural herbs, spices, vitamins, minerals, and antioxidants are required to reverse the damage. The following protocol is specific for the degree of damage suffered by the residents as a result of the trade center collapse: Beta carotene (natural source only) : 50,000 to 100,000 I.U. daily. Do this for two months, then reduce the amount to 25,000 I.U. daily. Be sure you take a 100% natural source of beta carotene.

Organic selenium: 600 to 800 mcg daily. Note: this must be the organic or amino acid bound type. Do not use sodium selenite or selenious acid. These synthetic types are potentially toxic.

Vitamin E: 800 I.U. daily (or, for a more powerful antioxidant action, take edible oil of wild rosemary, 10 drops twice daily).

Vitamin C: 1000 mg daily. Note: for optimal benefits also take crude natural sources of vitamin C, for instance, Flavin-C, four capsules twice daily.

Oreganol P73 oil of wild oregano: five to ten drops under the tongue twice daily. Take more if needed, like five to 10 drops four times daily. For difficult situations use the Super Strength oil of wild oregano at the same dosages.

Oregacyn: this is extremely valuable, ideal for reversing severe respiratory syndromes. Take one or two capsules twice daily. In the case of individuals working directly in the trade center environment and/or who have developed persistent lung symptoms, take larger amounts, like 2 or 3 capsules twice daily. Usually benefits are noted within days.

Respira Clenz is a multiple spice and herb oil extract with significant capacity to cleanse the lungs. Rich in natural antioxidants, this is ideal for reversing toxic lung damage. It also helps the lymphatic system extract, remove, and detoxify noxious agents, including germs, heavy metals, and hydrocarbons.

Vitamin C-rich foods are lung-friendly. Eat kiwi fruit, oranges, grapefruit, lemons, and limes as often as possible. Hot, spicy foods are also lung-friendly. Use cayenne, curry powder, horseradish, oregano, rosemary, cilantro, coriander, and similar spicy/hot substances. A recent USDA study (2002) proves that spices are by far the most powerful antioxidants. Incredibly, of all spices oregano was the most powerful. According to the USDA it "blew away" the competition. The oregano proved to be 40 times more powerful than apples and some 5 times more powerful than antioxidant-rich blueberries. Chicken soup made with large amounts of garlic and onion, as well as a teaspoon or two of wild oregano, helps clear and heal the lungs. Add plenty of nutrient-rich vegetables such as broccoli, Brussel's sprouts, cauliflower, spinach, red sweet peppers, and green peppers. Strictly avoid cigarette smoke. If you are a smoker, quit.

Flu

Globally, this is the most common cause of infectious epidemics. It causes a greater amount of misery, as well as death, than any other episodic infectious disease.

The flu is an extremely dangerous illness, in fact, its dangers are often underestimated. *The Chicago Tribune*, September 2001, offers stark evidence for its potential for devastation. According to the *Tribune* in 1918 the flu killed 100 million people globally. People fell dead quickly. No age group was immune but, surprisingly, 30 to 40 year old men, who would normally be resistant, were its greatest victims. This is the pandemic that today's experts fear. The number of victims could be astronomical: perhaps several hundred million. However, the more likely scenario is that, globally, between 20 to 80 million will die, still an incredibly large number. In the recent past the powers of a new strain of flu were felt. In 1957 the Asian flu killed 70,000 Americans.

The flu normally lasts only about three days to a week.

However, there has been developing a kind of increasing vulnerability to its toxicity. In certain instances it has lasted over 10 days, which may indicate that there is a weakening of the populations' immunity. Typically, the individual becomes exhausted and unable to function, suffering from aches, pains, nasal discharge and respiratory symptoms. Rarely, this leads to pneumonia, which may be fatal.

The source of the infection is usually contaminated air. Influenza spreads by droplets arising usually from human discharges. Sneezing and coughing liberates the virus on water droplets. It can live in this manner for at least 8 hours in the air. Thus, an epidemic is dependent upon the spread in civilized regions, where large numbers of people congregate. The original source is probably not man, but is, instead, swine. The virus flourishes in pig blood, and pigs excrete it in their urine, feces, and breath. Pork farms are the major site from which influenza spreads. This may explain why influenza often arises in China, where pork farms are common near populated regions.

The flu usually strikes suddenly. Symptoms can begin within 24 hours of exposure. It can spread fast. An entire family can succumb within a matter of hours. In fact, an entire community can succumb within days, perhaps hours.

With the flu there is always a danger for a global epidemic, which occurs approximately once every 35 years. The world is due for a severe epidemic.

The history of the pandemics is revealing. They have occurred in 1510, 1557, 1580, 1593, 1658, 1675, 1729, 1762, 1780, 1788, 1830, 1846, 1857, 1889, and 1918. As 1918 was the last time a pandemic occurred, it is long overdue and will likely occur around 2003 to 2005. When it occurs, it is possible that hundreds of thousands, perhaps millions, will die. Unless individuals are armed with the knowledge of potent natural cures, there will be little or no hope.

In severe cases complications occur. These include bacterial and fungal infections of the lungs, sinuses, ears, and mouth. Strep commonly attacks the weakened flu victim, as do molds and fungi. Thus, once the immune system is weakened by the flu virus the body is vulnerable to opportunistic infections. In some individuals a severe type of bronchitis may develop which may last for several days and greatly weaken the individual. In rare instances pneumonia develops, which may lead to death. In pandemics fatal pneumonia develops more frequently, causing a higher than usual death rate. The fact is influenza is one of the most dangerous of all infections, especially for the elderly

The flu may so greatly compromise immunity that the individual may fail to completely recover, or it may take weeks or months to regain strength. Bizarre side effects may develop, including kidney damage, nerve damage, paralysis, numbness, pink eye, iritis, visual loss, oral blisters, shingles, nerve damage, and even baldness.

Pigs spread human flu. A virus originating in swine, which mutated so that it could easily enter human cells, caused the 1918 flu. The pigs were immune, but humans had no immunity. Thus, the immune system was completely overwhelmed and failed to offer an adequate defense. Mark Gibbs of Australia's National University claims that researchers believe that the virus had infected pigs and then mutated, allowing it to aggressively invade humans.

Medically, there is nothing that can be done for the flu. The flu vaccine is virtually incompetent. The fact is there is no significant research proving efficacy or safety. It is fraught with side effects, including the serious paralysis condition known as Guillian-Barré syndrome. Even if it were effective, supplies are unreliable. Plus, there is no guarantee that the proper type of vaccine or sufficient quantities thereof will be available to defend against the crisis. Plus, vaccines are invariably vulnerable to being contaminated with germs, genetic material from germs, that is germ DNA, germ protein, and chemical preservatives, including mercury and aluminum. The individual must learn about and utilize natural cures if he/she wishes "guaranteed survival." This is because only natural substances offer virus-killing powers without damaging the immune system or other organs.

The book *Microbiology and Man*, written in 1949, provides invaluable information about what is the flu and how is it caused. Influenza is described as an acute infection which strikes suddenly, with it lasting from one to seven days. The common symptoms haven't changed: achiness, fatigue, exhaustion, pains in the back and limbs, nasal discharge, and respiratory symptoms. Uncomplicated cases are usually mild, but they may greatly weaken the individual. This may lead to future disease or even a sudden bout of potentially fatal pneumonia. These early authors remind us that influenza may be elusive, that is the symptoms are so vague that it may not be correctly diagnosed. This may prove dangerous, because the flu must be taken seriously, and the proper treatment and precautions must be urgently administered.

The older theories regarding the cause of influenza are fascinating and are certainly accurate. The frank cause is a virus. However, early studies found that a bacteria is associated, the throat germ known as *Hemophilus influenzae.* This germ apparently contributes to the illness but, obviously, the virus is the primary culprit. Apparently, the virus lives and reproduces in this bacteria.

The role of other germs, like Hemophilus, is exemplified by the infectious history in the main reservoir for the flu virus: hogs. In Iowa in 1918 a disease appeared in hogs which was so similar to the human flu that it was promptly named "swine flu." The disease, which is exceedingly lethal, strikes a herd in the same way the flu virus strikes human groups. In 1931 Richard Shope of the Rockefeller Institute in a series of well designed investigations in pigs showed that the disease was due to a virus and that a bacteria, the *Hemophilus influenza*, was also a player. Dr. Shope found that it was necessary for both germs to be present to cause severe flu.

This is how the virus and bacteria, at least in hogs, are related. Swine flu usually only occurs from October to December. Shope found that the Hemophilus germ, which is needed to produce the disease in hogs, was present all year, primarily in the nasal and respiratory passages. In contrast, the virus is only in swine seasonally. Since viruses cannot survive without infecting, that is parasitizing, cells, they are rarely permanent residents and are usually cleared by the immune system from the tissues, or they enter into a form of hibernation. He was originally unable to determine where the virus went in the remaining months, in other words, it couldn't just appear out of nowhere. It had to have a host. Shope suspected that there must be another agent, a parasite which keeps the virus viable. He found two such parasites, both of them worms. One was the hog lungworm, and the other, incredibly, was the common earthworm. This is how transmission and infectivity are maintained.

During the acute flu infection the hog lungworm becomes infected with the virus. These are coughed up, swallowed, and excreted in the feces. The residue in the feces is eaten by the earthworm, which acts as a host. In other words, the eggs of the hog worm actually hatch within the earthworm, living off of it. The hog then eats the earthworms, and the cycle continues endlessly. When the earthworms are digested, the lungworm's eggs, infected with flu virus, are liberated, ultimately reaching the lungs, where they develop into worms. Yet, for whatever reason, this is not sufficient to provoke severe flu unless the bacteria *Hemophilus influenza* (swine variety) is present. Thus, the hog, laden with various parasites, harbors and maintains the very germ which has the potential of causing millions of deaths globally.

Treatment protocol

For mild cases take the multi-spice antiseptic formula, that is the Oregacyn, 2 to 3 capsules three times daily. For tough cases take it more often, as much as a capsule or two every hour. There is no toxicity, since it is made from edible and wild spices. For prevention take one or two capsules daily. For additional power take the oil of wild oregano (Oreganol), 2 to 5 drops under the tongue several times daily. Continue until symptoms disappear. For tough cases the key is rapidity; it may be necessary to take it every few minutes until symptoms clear. Wild oregano is an absolute cure for influenza. For additional power take the highly antiviral Oregacyn, either as capsules or as Oregacyn oil. With the capsules take one or two every four hours. With the oil take a few drops under the tongue every hour. Avoid the consumption of pork, including ham, bacon, sausage, pepperoni, bologna, etc. Also, do not eat or drink food containing refined sugar. High doses may require the intake of healthy bacteria, that is probiotic supplements. For ideal results take such supplements right before bedtime. (Health Bac)

Hay fever

This is one of the most commonly occurring of all allergic diseases, afflicting tens of millions of North Americans. It mainly attacks the nose and eyes, causing congestion, sneezing, and nasal drainage.

The term hay fever is misleading. Usually, there is no fever. Plus, hay is only one of many hundreds of protein/pollen sources which may provoke it. However, the "hay" portion of the name is revealing: wet hay is a source of various pollens, as well as molds, and reactions to it by farmers and other individuals working closely with hay may have initiated the name. The fact is wet hay breeds molds, and these molds produced untold billions of spores, which may be liberated in hot or windy weather. Thus, a more correct name would be moldy hay fever.

Hay fever can cause a great deal of misery, even though it is not serious. However, the discomfort, which includes obstructed breathing, sneezing, watery eyes, itching of the eyes/nose, and nasal discharge, is serious, since it significantly affects lifestyle.

Hay fever is usually most severe during August and September, finally ending at the first frost. The fact that it ends at this time is a clear indication of the role of molds as a major cause, since cold weather distroys them. There is also a spring type due to tree pollens and the pollens of certain grasses. Obviously, the risks are greatest when the pollen counts are high. This is also the time when mold counts are highest. Thus the symptoms of hay fever are due to a reaction against both pollens and molds. However, at the root of this is a rarely recognized fact, that is that there may be an underlying chronic sinus or lung infection, which makes the individual more vulnerable to the hay fever allergens. Mold/yeast infestation is the usual cause of this undiagnosed infection. Such individuals may react violently when the mold counts in the air rise.

Pollen is an outdoor substance; the counts indoors are comparatively low. Staying indoors in an air conditioned home is one rather extreme therapy. Pollen counts are also low in the mountains or seaside. Incredibly, there is no truly pollen-free region, except, perhaps, the far north of Canada. Even so, doctors may recommend that a sufferer visit the seaside or the high mountains as a therapy. What's more, the seashore offers relief only when the wind is blowing in from the ocean. However, this is a rather extreme therapy. Fortunately, there is a solution for correcting this distressing condition without leaving your home.

The medical treatment for hay fever is essentially nonexistent. There are no drugs which cure it, only a few, such as antihistamines, modify symptoms. A specialized therapy known as "desensitization" may be offered. However, this is both painful and cumbersome and only occasionally offers a cure. Thus, natural remedies are the only solutions.

Treatment protocol

Crude extracts of wild medicinal spices offer significant anti-histaminic and anti-mold actions. Spice and herb extracts offer safety unavailable from over-the-counter agents.

Certain spice extracts, notably oil of oregano, clove, sage, and bay leaf, offer potent antihistaminic actions. What's more, they are antifungal powers. Thus, they are the ideal tonics for reversing this condition. Also, oil of wild oregano, taken under the tongue, can be an effective treatment for rapidly halting the symptoms of this condition. Take Oregacyn, which contains multiple antihistaminic spices, one or two capsules as needed. Also, take oil of wild oregano, a few drops under the tongue as needed. Citrus bioflavonoids are antihistaminic; take Flavin-C, bioflavonoid formula, three capsules twice or more daily.

Histoplasmosis

This is a rather serious lung infection caused by a fungus. This type of fungus most commonly grows in moist climates, especially in river valleys. Areas where birds congregate are another hot spot, because bird droppings cause the fungus to flourish. In the Ohio and Mississippi river valleys the infection is common. Thousands, perhaps millions, of people may have the infection and be unaware of it. Incredibly, according to the National Tuberculosis and Respiratory Disease Association as many as 50 million Americans unknowingly suffer from histoplasmosis.

Children are particularly vulnerable to this infection and for some unknown reason males are more commonly affected than females. In fact, the ratio is seven to one. In the Midwest there are also millions of males who unknowingly suffer the infection. The common Midwestern "summer/fall flu" may in fact be a fungal infection in the form of histoplasmosis. The only difference between the flu is that histoplasmosis may last for weeks, and it may take weeks or months to recover. Chest X-rays may reveal that what was thought to be the flu is a persistent fungal lung infection. However, even if the chest X-rays are negative this fails to rule out histoplasmosis, since in its early stages medical testing may be equivocal.

The fungus attacks the lymphatic system, as well as the liver and spleen, causing enlargement of these organs. However, the lungs suffer the brunt of the damage, and this is how doctors usually discover it, that is they see evidence of it on X-ray.

Histoplasmosis is an aggressive organism. It attacks a wide range of organs, particularly the liver, spleen, lungs, lymph nodes, bone marrow, adrenals, and intestines. It even invades the white blood cells and may thereby evade the immune system.

Treatment protocol

Take a multiple-spice extract, such as Oregacyn, 2 or 3 capsules twice daily. Take also Oreganol, 10 drops under the tongue twice daily. To further cleanse the lungs of pathogens and improve blood flow to the lungs take Respira Clenz, 10 to 20 drops twice daily. Also, increase the intake of foods rich in essential fatty acids. The essential fatty acids strengthen immunity and help increase the resistance against fungal infections. Take primrose oil, 6 capsules twice daily. Selenium is protective against lung fungal infections. The regular intake of this mineral assists the immune system in preventing the colonization by fungi. Take organically bound selenium, about 400 mcg daily.

Nasal polyps

This condition is caused by the hypertrophy of the mucous membranes of the lining of the nose. According to *Dorland's Medical Dictionary* nasal polyps are a type of tumor.

Nasal polyps are evidence of the existence of irritants. The irritants may be chemical or microbial. For instance, viral infections may induce them. What's more, they are a sign of nutritional imbalances. Deficiencies of vitamins A and C have been associated with the development of polyps. In fact, some texts describe them as a deliberate sign of vitamin A deficiency. The deficiency of these vitamins as a cause makes sense, because both vitamins A and C are needed to protect the mucous membranes against toxicity as well as viral infection.

Nasal polyps can become sufficient in size to cause obstruction in breathing. In this respect they can prove dangerous. Polyps may also develop as a consequence of drug therapy. Despite this fact drugs are the common treatment. Yet, since the polyps are caused largely by nutritional deficiency, as well as viral infection, the drugs fail to treat the cause and, thus, usually fail to correct it.

Treatment should include a diet high in vitamin A- and C-rich foods. Ideal food sources of vitamin A include organic liver, squash, sweet potatoes, sardines, salmon, egg yolk, and dark green leafy vegetables. Excellent sources of natural vitamin C include citrus fruit, guava, papaya, kiwi, citrus juice, lemons, limes, unsweetened currant juice, spinach, and broccoli. Refined sugar and flour should be completely avoided. All alcoholic beverages must be avoided. If you smoke, quit.

Treatment protocol

As a vitamin A source eat a can or two of sardines daily. Also, eat organic calf's or lamb's liver at least twice weekly. Take oil of wild oregano, five drops sublingually twice daily. Also, take Oregacyn, one or two capsules twice daily. As a source of crude unprocessed natural vitamin C take Flavin-C, three capsules twice daily. Flavin-C contains antiinflammatory bioflavonoids, which help decrease the swelling of the polyps and prevent recurrence. Also, take a vitamin A supplement, about 10,000 I.U. daily.

Pleurisy

This pneumonia-like condition is due to inflammation of the linings of the lungs, that is the pleura. It often occurs as a secondary effect to pneumonia. It may also be a sign of tuberculosis. The fact is a sudden case of pleurisy where no other cause is obvious often warns of hidden TB.

In this condition the individual is afflicted with the sudden onset of a very sharp pain, like a stabbing pain. The pain occurs with every breath. Coughing causes severe stabbing pain. Usually, there is high fever and chills as well as aches and pains. Bacteria are a primary cause, but fungi and molds can also provoke it.

Bacteria can cause severe inflammation, leading to scar formation. The inflammation and scarring causes the pleuritic pain. Treatment should be aimed not only at eradicating he germs but also at the reversal of the inflammation, plus the breakdown of the scarring.

Treatment protocol

Bacteria and molds, the major causes of pleurisy, quickly succumb to the powers of multiple spice extracts. Certain of the extracts, such as extracts of wild oregano and cloves, exhibit significant pain-killing powers. Take Oregacyn, the multiple edible spice extract, 2 capsules three or more times daily. Take a few extra capsules whenever the pain strikes. Rub P73 oil of wild oregano over the ribs and on the mid-back as often as necessary. Take 2 or more drops of the oil under the tongue two or more times daily. To digest the scars and reduce inflammation take the protein-digesting plant enzymes concentrate, that is BromaZyme, 3 or 4 capsules twice daily on an empty stomach. Also, take the antiinflammatory citrus bioflavonoid complex, Flavin-C, 4 or more capsules twice daily on an empty stomach.

Hot tea can help relieve the pain, especially if hot spices are added. Chop or slice fresh ginger root, and add to your favorite hot herbal tea. Clove buds may also be added. Drink several cups daily.

Pneumonia

This is one of the most serious of all respiratory illnesses. Usually, it is caused by a bacteria known descriptively as pneumococcus. This germ normally lives in the nose, sinuses, and throat. If it does get into the lungs, in the normal individual, it is rapidly destroyed. However, if the immune system is compromised, the germ may overgrow, causing severe infection and inflammation. This most commonly occurs in the weak and debilitated. Hospitalized patients, especially those with cancer or AIDS, are the most vulnerable to developing this serious disease. In fact, pneumonia is the primary cause of death in these individuals.

Pneumonia is usually a secondary effect of other conditions. For instance, let's say an elderly but healthy person has a hip fracture. This results in stress and immobility. The individual is hospitalized in a weakened state. Hospital food is notoriously poor, which further compromises resistance. Pneumonia develops and, often, kills the individual. Hospitalized cancer patients often suffer the same fate. Their resistance is compromised, plus they are often undergoing toxic therapies, such as radiation or chemotherapy, which greatly depress immunity. When the powers of the immune system decline, the lungs are easily colonized by a host of pathogens, such as Candida albicans, pneumococcus, staph, or various parasites, and the individual rapidly succumbs. Drug resistant highly pathogenic germs abound in hospital enviroments. These germs aggressively attack and invade the human body. There is far less risk for fatal pneumonia in cancer patients treated outside of the hospital.

Hospitals house a vast number of pathogens, many of which are freaks of nature. These biochemical freaks are the consequence of the overuse of antibiotics and are known medically as mutant bacteria. The mutants cause frighteningly severe infections, which rapidly induce fatality, plus there are no medical cures against them.

Treatment protocol

Be sure the room is well ventilated; do not be afraid of opening windows. Be sure to open them fully. Plenty of rest is necessary. The room should be quiet: no television or radio should be allowed. Soft music may be played, however, in general, quiet time is needed for healing. Anyone entering the room must be sure to wash the hands before touching the victim. Also, be sure to wash the hands thoroughly after touching. Hot herbal teas are the drink of choice along with freshly squeezed grapefruit or orange juice. Curtail the intake of coffee and black tea.

Chocolate and sugar should be avoided. The diet should be free of all milk products. Little food should be eaten. Clear beef or chicken broth soups are the ideal nourishment along with fresh fruit and/or vegetables. During severe infections heavy meals rich in protein interfere with the healing process. The patient should eat lightly: fruit, soups, broths, and fruit or vegetable juices only. The air should be cleansed with essential oils. In a spray bottle add hot water along with oils of bay leaf, oregano, rosemary, and lavender, or use the Germ-A-Clenz. pump spray. Shake well and pump spray the room. Repeat a few times daily until the condition is resolved. Take Oregacyn, two or more capsules three times daily. Also, take oil of wild Oreganol, 10 or more drops several times daily. For severe cases take it more often, like every hour.

Sarcoidosis

This condition is officially listed as due to unknown causes. Yet, certainly, infection is the likely cause, and fungi and/or yeasts are the probable culprits. Sarcoidosis attacks the entire body, however, the lungs are the main site of infestation.

The disease is regional, occurring mainly in the South, particularly in areas which have a humid climate, like the Carolinas, Georgia, Alabama, Mississippi, Kentucky, Virginia, and Florida. Incredibly, in Europe Sweden and Norway have the highest incidence. There is also a racial propensity. For some unknown reason people of African descent are 10 times more likely to develop it than Caucasians.

The disease is manifested by sarcoids, which are lesions in the lungs, lymph nodes, and skin. There may be hundreds of these lesions in the lungs. These lesions induce inflammation and scarring. This is why cortisone is frequently prescribed. Sarcoidosis often is discovered due to the existence of skin lesions and/or swollen lymph glands.

Treatment protocol

Fungus is the most likely cause of sarcoidosis. Currently, the type of fungus is unknown. The fact that fungus is the obvious cause becomes readily apparent by how and where it develops. Sarcoidosis occurs mainly in the Deep South, where humidity and mold counts are particularly high. The fungal cause is also revealed by the fact that it has a propensity to attack the lungs, the region of the body most vulnerable to fungal invasion. This is why antifungal spice extracts are the ideal treatment. Such extracts kill the entire range of molds, fungi, and yeasts. Plus, they exhibit significant antiinflammatory properties. To reverse this condition take Oregacyn, two or more capsules twice daily. Natural antiinflammatory agents are indicated. Take BromaZyme, a combination of papain and bromelain, 3 capsules twice daily on an empty stomach. Also, take crude natural bioflavonoids, such as Flavin-C, 3 or more capsules daily. The combination of enzymes plus bioflavonoids offers significant antiinflammatory powers, without side effects.

Scoliosis and Pott's disease: the hunch back syndromes

Neurologically, the lungs are one of the most sensitive of all organs. They are supplied by hundreds of miles of nerves. These nerves arise mainly from the spinal cord, although a few arise directly from the brain. Nerves control lung function. If they are irritated, the lungs are also irritated. Incredibly, this also happens in reverse: if the lungs are irritated, they send messages through the nerves to the spine and ultimately the spinal muscles. This may lead to a condition known as spinal atrophy, which means that the muscles degenerate.

Scoliosis and hunch back, that is kyphosis of the spine, are consequences of lung disease. The lungs lie directly behind the spine. If they are diseased, they send messages via the nervous system to the spine. These messages cause stress, leading to destruction of the bones and joints. Thus, in many instances a twisted and bowed back may not be primarily a spinal defect, that is the defect arises mainly within the body, specifically the lungs. Thus, in order to cure the deformity or prevent it from worsening the lungs must be cleansed of all invaders as well as toxins.

The spine is one of the most important organs of the body. Normally, it is straight, that is it doesn't deviate from the midline. It has certain normal curvatures within this up and down structure. These are found in the neck, mid back, and lower lumbar regions. However, any degree of lateral or side-ways curvature is abnormal. This is known as scoliosis. This sideways curvature develops directly over the lung reflexes, that is the region of the spine supplied by the lungs' nerves. Scoliosis is pathological, and the likely site of the pathology is the lung.

Chronic infections of the lungs may be difficult to diagnose, and, thus, in an individual with scoliosis this lung component may have never been considered as a cause. It is not the only cause. A severe deficiency of nutrients, particularly vitamin D and calcium, may result in scoliosis. Other minerals are needed for bone formation, particularly zinc and magnesium. Vitamin A is also needed for the creation of healthy bone. Thus, individuals who are poorly nourished or who had poor nourishment in utero may develop this disorder. However, it is crucial to consider the infection connection. The infection may be hidden in the lungs, but it is also often disguised in the sinuses, tonsils, or adenoids or even the teeth.

Scoliosis may develop suddenly, usually after a severe infection. Other regions besides the lungs may be involved. Infections in the intestines, tonsils, ears, and adenoids have all been known to cause it. Tuberculosis is also a major cause. This may be a hidden cause, that is a low-grade type of tuberculosis that defies diagnosis. Yet, in a frail-appearing child, teenager, or young adult who develops scoliosis, the diagnosis of tuberculosis must be high on the list. This is especially true of the individual who is poorly nourished, of dark-skinned nature, and/or who fails to get sufficient sunshine.

Constipation has also been recognized as a cause. This may be due to the fact that toxins in the colon may be absorbed into the blood, poisoning lung tissue. The lung tissue acts as a sieve, absorbing toxins from the blood much like a living sponge. Cleansing of the colon may rapidly result in an improvement, even helping to induce a straightening of the spine. However, the cleansing program must be consistent, because if the toxic condition returns, the scoliosis worsens.

The germ that causes tuberculosis is a slow growing organism. Thus, it may be impossible to diagnose by cultures or blood tests. Plus, there are few if any reliable ways to discover its presence. Thus, symptoms and signs, that is obvious physical damage, can be relied upon to make the diagnosis. With the exception of that caused by obvious injury a deformed or crooked spine in a youngster or young adult is a clear indication of chronic tuberculosis. There is not only deformity but also chronic pain. The most prominent symptom of undiagnosed spinal tuberculosis is pain, which may be felt in many areas. It could be a type of hip pain or possibly sciatica, that is pain down the back of the leg or hip. A vague type of abdominal pain that defies diagnosis may also represent tuberculosis. Spinal stiffness, including ankylosing spondylitis, may be merely a representation of internal tubercular infection. Both the bones of the spinal column and the discs between the vertebrae are readily infected. However, even if the infection is in other regions, like within the lungs or abdominal cavity, it may lead to scoliosis, spinal stiffness, or other spinal deformities. This is because tubercular infection causes massive scarring, which drags the vertebrae out of alignment. However, pain and deformity are only a few of the key symptoms of TB. Other common symptoms include in the early stages low body temperature in the morning, slight fever, especially in the afternoon, weight loss, slight persistent cough, history of exposure (from humans or contaminated food) and, later, persistent fever, chronic cough, coughing of blood or sputum, and increasing weight loss. Fistulas are another important sign. Fulminant night sweats may also be an indicator.

Nutritional deficiency plays an enormous role in scoliosis. This is because deficiencies of amino acids, vitamins, minerals, and fatty acids greatly weaken immunity, increasing the risks for the development of chronic infection. Plus, the deficiencies cause a weakening of connective tissues. This weakening allows various germs to gain entry into the tissues, causing chronic infection. In tuberculosis and/or scoliosis dozens of nutrients are usually severely lacking. However, the primary deficiencies include a lack of amino acids, vitamin A, vitamin D, riboflavin, pantothenic acid, magnesium, zinc, and, particularly, vitamin C. The fact is a chronic lack of vitamin C greatly increases the risk for the development of both scoliosis and tuberculosis.

In all cases of rigidity of the spine tuberculosis must be considered. Other infections may also be the cause such as Lyme, staph, or candida. In this instance the normal curves of the spine disappear, a condition which may be described as "poker-back." This is due to inflammation in the joints. The inflammation results from infection. There are many sites for the infection, including the spinal column itself, the teeth, liver, spleen, intestines, sinuses, and blood.

Treatment protocol

Tuberculosis, scoliosis, and spinal deformity require aggressive therapy. It may require a prolonged period of supplementation, such as several months, to reverse such disorders.

Massage and osteopathic treatments are of enormous benefit. The diet must be rich in highly nutritious foods. Only nutrient dense foods must be consumed. The foods with the greatest nutrient density include eggs, whole milk products, cheese, red meat, poultry, fish, fresh fruit, and fresh vegetables. What's more, the intake of fresh whole organic milk is critical. The protein in milk greatly aids in boosting immunity. The exception is the individual who is allergic to it. In this instance consume fresh whole milk yogurt or perhaps goat's milk. Milk is also rich in riboflavin, which is needed for oxygen metabolism. Riboflavin aids in the prevention and reversal of TB: oxygen is toxic to this germ. If the riboflavin content of the lungs is high, so will be the oxygen utilization potential. Thus, a diet rich in riboflavin may act as a tuberculosis preventive. For more information in assessing your level of riboflavin and/or vitamin deficiencies see the Web site, Nutritiontest.com. During the 1920s whole milk, rich in riboflavin, was an essential component for reversing TB.

A natural vegetable source of riboflavin in a concentrated form is available. Known as Wild Green Powerdrops, these drops are made exclusively from unprocessed wild greens. Therefore, they are completely different than the commercial greens and, thus, far more powerful. Plus, they contain wild nettle extract, invaluable for promoting healthy lungs. As a tonic and natural source of the lung nourishing riboflavin, take 20 or more drops twice daily. This is a rare nutritional supplement: only a limited amount is available yearly, since it is picked totally from the wild by specially trained bushmen.

Milk still remains a mainstay in tuberculosis treatment. However, today, the milk is less nutritious than it was in the past. If fresh whole milk is available, it should be consumed on a daily basis. In sanatoriums fresh whole milk directly from cows or goats was fed to TB victims with tremendous results. For more information about the healing powers of fresh whole milk and other nutrient dense foods see the books, *Lifesaving Cures and How to Eat Right and Live Longer.*

Silicosis (silica deposits in the lungs)

This is perhaps the most frequent work-related disease of the lungs caused by industrial particles. Silica particles are highly toxic to lung tissue and cause severe scarring. When the lung tissues become scarred, they are weakened and, thus, these tissues become vulnerable to infection. In fact, tuberculosis is a common consequence of silicosis. So is chronic bronchitis.

The fact is certain cases may present as the latter and, thus, be erroneously treated with antibiotics, cortisone, etc. What's more, occasionally silicosis may be misdiagnosed as asthma.

Silicosis is common in miners and also individuals who work in the sandblasting, concrete, demolition, and stone polishing industries. While it was an epidemic in such workers in the past, today, precautions have been taken which reduce the risks. Obviously, the greatest precaution is wearing protective masks. Silicosis may be one of the complications being experienced by people in New York exposed to the Trade Center dust.

The symptoms of silicosis are rather vague and may mimic many other lung disorders, including bronchitis, emphysema, and asthma. It begins with shortness of breath, worsened by exertion. Wheezing and coughing usually follow, along with a weakening of the resistance against respiratory infections. As it worsens, sputum, which is grey colored or blood stained, may be produced. The final stage includes coughing of blood, which warns of tuberculosis. Chest X-rays may mimic the typical barrel chest of emphysema and, of course, reveal the characteristic silica nodules.

When the silica dust is inhaled, it is lodged in the deep recesses of the lungs. There, it is attacked by white blood cells, which attempt to remove it through the lymph. The white blood cells, as well as the lung's lymphatic glands, attempt to detoxify or destroy the silica. However, silica is a hard mineral and is difficult to decompose. Eventually, it plugs the lymphatics, leading to scarring. Thus, therapy must be aimed at stimulating the flow of lymph and preventing further scarring. What's more, efforts should be made to break down the scars through enzyme therapy as well as the inhalation of the appropriate essential oils.

If no treatment is given, the condition gradually worsens. Eventually, nodules filled with silica become visible on X-ray. The entire lung may eventually become fibrotic, and death usually occurs from infections, often tuberculous. This is where nature offers the most productive answers, since there is no medical cure for silicosis.

Essential oils, particularly spice oils, are an ideal therapy for this condition. Such oils act as solvents, denuding the silica molecules, essentially dissolving them. In other words, they cause the silica to be rendered water soluble. Spice oils offer the additional benefit of being antimicrobial. Italian research indicates that spice oils are actually able to dissolve silica deposits. Oils of wild oregano, rosemary, clove, cinnamon, and sage are all ideal for reversing this condition. Many of these oils are available in formulas, that is Respira Clenz and Oregacyn, which are multiple spice extracts.

Treatment protocol

Dust is the carrier for this disease, and that is where the danger is. The simplest treatment is avoidance, that is taking precautions to avoid or minimize inhalation of the dust. This means wearing the appropriate masks at all times. Massive efforts must be made to help the body extract or dissolve the silica deposits. This may be a monumental task; however, it is not insurmountable. In order to dissolve scar tissue take BromaZyme, 2 or 3 capsules three times daily on an empty stomach. This contains a potent type of fruit enzyme capable of dissolving scar tissue. Also, take vitamin E, 400 I. U. daily. Essential oils have solvent properties, and, thus, they help dissolve organic compounds, including silica deposits. Oils of oregano, rosemary, sage, cloves, and juniper all exhibit these properties. Take P73 oil of wild oregano (SuperStrength variety is the best), five to ten drops twice daily. Also, take a special combination of these oils, Respira Clenz, 20 drops twice daily. This is highly respected by doctors as an effective agent for lung support. For additional power take the multiple spice extract, that is Oregacyn, two capsules twice daily. Crude wild greens also assist lung function. Take the Wild Green powerdrops, 20 drops twice daily. The latter is high in natural riboflavin, which is needed for oxygen transport in the lungs. The wild greens is a rare nutritional supplement and is not available in stores. To order call 1-800-243-5242.

Sinusitis

This is one of modern humankind's greatest epidemics. Sinusitis afflicts tens of millions of North Americans. It is usually a chronic ailment, seemingly unresponsive to any type of medication. It may be defined as inflammation and/or swelling in the sinuses. These toxic effects are usually caused by infection.

The sinuses, along with the nasal passages, are a key organ of respiration. Both the nose and the sinuses act as radiators, warming the air. They also act as filters, removing particles that could severely damage the lungs. As a sort of air conditioner, they add moisture to the air, as necessary, since air which is too dry may also damage the lungs. The nasal and sinus membranes produce mucous, which is a key secretion for protecting the lungs from toxicity. This mucous helps trap harmful particles, as well as germs, so they may be detoxified and/or destroyed. Thus, in essence the nose and sinuses are a sort of house cleaner for the lungs, keeping these organs from being burdened by harmful agents.

The cilia are a fascinating organ system found within the nasal and sinus regions. These are delicate hair-like organs, but they are not stiff or coarse. They are delicate like tiny velvet fibers. Their job is to cleanse the mucous, acting essentially like a living conveyor belt. They constantly push inhaled "garbage" towards the stomach, so that it cannot go into the lungs.

There are several sinus cavities. Some are located just above the eyes on the lower forehead. Others are located just under the cheekbone. Yet, others are located on either side of the nose and behind the nose deep in the facial bones.

Sinus disorders may exhibit a wide range of symptoms. The symptoms are so diverse and/or bizarre that the proper diagnosis is frequently missed. Headache is perhaps the most common symptom, along with pressure in the face or forehead. Stuffiness of the nose is also a signal. Post nasal drip may indicate the existence of chronic sinus infection and/or allergy. Also, there is often the complaint of thick mucous at the back of the throat that simply cannot be cleared. Facial pain may have its primary origin in sinus infection as well as pain in the teeth. Common patterns of pain include pain over one eye, generalized head pain, one-sided headache, pain on the tip of the head, pain in the ear, neck pain, pain between the shoulder blades, and arm pain. Infection or inflammation in the sphenoid sinus, which is located behind the nose fairly close to the inner ear, may create symptoms in the ear. Dr. Albert Seltzer, sinus specialist, describes a case of a woman who complained of noises in her ear, sounding like a foghorn or at other times like a whistle. Treating the sinus disorder cured the symptoms.

Even colds may have their origin in sinus problems, especially in the person who suffers from repeated bouts. Dr. Seltzer describes another odd case: a person complaining of dark spots before the eyes. When the sinus infection was cured, the eye problems disappeared. It is easy to comprehend from the diversity of symptoms why the diagnosis is often elusive.

Traditionally, bacterial infections have been regarded as the primary cause of sinusitis. Yet, antibiotics have been found to be largely ineffective. This is because the model for the treatment of sinus disorders has been erroneous. Mayo Clinic recently proved this. Doctors at the Clinic were stymied as to why sinus patients failed to improve despite intensive antibiotic therapy. They cultured the sinuses and failed to find bacteria. Instead, they found molds. In fact, 40 different molds and yeasts were recovered. Their conclusion was that chronic sinus disease is due to fungal infection. Antibiotics are useless against fungi, in fact, these drugs enhance fungal growth.

Dental disorders may lead to sinus infections. The upper teeth are directly connected to the roof of the sinuses. If the teeth are infected, the toxins and germs readily enter the sinuses, causing a wide range of symptoms. Some of the more prominent symptoms include stuffy sinuses, sinus drainage, sinus headaches, facial pain, pain around the eye, and even seemingly remote symptoms, like arm, hip, leg, and back pain. Dr. Seltzer describes numerous cases where when the dental problems were cured, the sinus problems completely disappeared.

Sinus disorders may arise after flying. This is caused by the tremendous forces resulting from pressure changes in the ears, most prominently occurring during takeoff and landing. The eustachian tube between the nose and ears attempts to equalize the pressure so that it won't damage the head, that is the brain. The pressure changes that occur within this tube lead to swelling, or they may force nasal or sinus secretions deeper into the sinuses or even into the inner ear. If secretions enter the inner ear, infection may develop. In adults this infection has been known to cause hearing loss: even deafness.

Treatment protocol

Oregacyn is a potent therapy for sinusitis. It helps halt excessive secretions while destroying noxious microbes. To correct this problem take one to two capsules twice daily. For difficult problems take more, like 3 or 4 capsules three times daily. This dosage is acceptable for 2 weeks, then reduce it to 1 to 4 capsules daily. Also, take oil of wild oregano, five or more drops twice daily. For difficult conditions increase the dosage. The oil may also be rubbed on the sinus regions, like the forehead or under the cheek bones. Or, it may be inhaled directly. Extremely difficult conditions may require the use of the SuperStrength oil of wild oregano. Take ten or more drops twice daily under the tongue. After placing it under the tongue, hold it against the tissues with the tip of the tongue for at least a minute. This will aid in penetration, because under the tongue administration gets the oil directly into the blood. If flying, be sure to take an Oregacyn just before take-off and another capsule just before landing.

Smallpox

This disease is caused by a virus known medically as the variola virus. This virus is the largest known to infect humans.

While it is large compared to other viruses, it is still tiny by microbial standards. Some three million smallpox viruses fit on the tip of a pen.

From pictures it would appear that smallpox is a skin disease. This is misleading, because, while there are obvious skin lesions, it has a viscous effect upon the entire body, including the internal organs.

Historically, smallpox was perhaps the most feared, as well as common, of all communicable diseases. It is the greatest infectious killer of all time. In fact, it is such an aggressive killer that it altered the course of the Roman Empire, accelerating its decline. It also changed the course of history in America. The Native Americans, who had no immunity to it, were largely destroyed by this disease. They were victims of biological warfare. Europeans, notably the Englishman, Sir Jeffrey Amhurst, deliberately introduced the virus into native communities. He did so by sending them the "gift" of smallpox infested blankets, that is blankets used by smallpox victims. As a result, millions of natives died, making the conquering of their race far easier. The Europeans had sufficient history of exposure and, therefore, immunity, while the natives, a virgin population, had no immunity. In some regions 90% of the native population was destroyed. This lead to the rapid expansion of Western civilization.

It is a scary disease, also because of what it does cosmetically to the body. It may cause permanent scarring, especially on the face and torso. It is also feared, because of the intense pain and misery it causes. When it strikes, people become totally bedridden. Plus, they experience severe pain and a bizarre burning sensation on the skin and mucous membranes.

Smallpox is currently extinct in the United States and other Western countries. In fact, it has apparently been eradicated globally. However, stores of smallpox germs exist in microbiological labs, where they are stored for research or as potential biological agents. Thus, if a deliberate attempt were made to seed this virus, a localized or even global epidemic could occur.

When smallpox strikes, it is particularly dangerous for children as well as the fetus. Here, it is highly fatal. However, with adults the fatality rate is also high: some 30%. Blacks are unusually susceptible, as are Native Americans. However, currently, virtually everyone globally, especially Westerners, is highly vulnerable.

The germ gains entrance into the body through the lungs: thus, sneezing, breathing, and coughing mainly disseminate it. Merely talking could transmit it. However, there are few obvious lung signs. Rather, the obvious signs are in the skin and mucous membranes. Pustules occur on the skin, and ulcers appear on the mucous membranes. The skin may suffer tiny hemorrhages. The skin lesions may become boil-like, and they may coalesce into large boil-like patches. The lungs usually only become symptomatic as the result of secondary bacterial infections. As the infection extends the internal organs may swell and hemorrhage. If the internal swelling and hemorrhaging becomes extreme, death may rapidly ensue.

The existence of infection may not be readily evident. This is because smallpox has a relatively long incubation period: about 15 days. When it does initiate, it may begin with chills, utter exhaustion, prostration (can't get out of the bed), skin boils and pustules, which tend to grow bigger and eventually touch each other, severe pain, and fever. Regarding the latter the fever rapidly rises, and then gradually falls. The fever can be extreme: up to 107 degrees. As it falls the skin eruptions occur. The eruptions begin as pimples, then boils, then pus pimples (pustule), and then crusted lesions. As described in T. J. Ritter, M. D., in *Mother's Remedies*, published in 1910, any non-vacinnated person who is exposed will contract this dreaded disease.

However, mass vaccinations are not without risk. The sudden and unbridled imposition of vaccinations in the entire populous could lead to a wide range of ill effects: even thousands of deaths. The authorities who promote such mass vaccinations rarely if ever expose the untoward effects. This is because the attitude taken regarding mass vaccinations is that what is supposedly good for humanity at large is worth any risk, that is the risk for side effects and loss of life. However, this is merely advertising jargon: no evidence is provided of a scientifically proven benefit. What's more, the production of vaccinations is an enormous business. Thus, vested interests promote vaccinations for financial gain. In fact, billions stand to be made, literally overnight, if national vaccination programs are ordained. Even so, it is true that direct exposure is the most risky type. This is because the smallpox vesicles are highly infective. Thus, special precautions must be taken in order to prevent the spread of this disease. Here is where essential oils prove of enormous value. They offer significant antiseptic actions, both in the air and on or in the body.

What's more, there is no certain evidence that vaccinations cure or prevent the disease. In the Western world the incidence declines in concert with improvements in sanitation, that is improved housing, reduction of poverty, chlorination of water, proper disposal of garbage, improved food supply, etc. According to J. H. Greer, M.D., author of *A Physician in the House*, in the United States smallpox was known as a "filth disease", one propagated by unsanitary conditions. The fact is it was largely a disease of the poor and lower class, and it was routinely fatal in the impoverished and/or malnourished, that is where there was poor attention to proper cleanliness and hygiene. Thus, in the current global climate smallpox is likely to make a comeback, since there has been a vast dilemma of global strife, war, and poverty, as well as the war-induced destruction of infrastructure, sanitation, etc. The fact is this is the ideal climate for the regeneration of this disease. What's more, apparently, outbreaks are being reported in the war-torn regions of the former Yugoslavia. Afghanistan, replete with sanitation-poor refugee camps, is yet another likely climate for the outbreak.

Dr. Greer continues that proper sanitation was only a 20th century science. He provides compelling proof that the sanitation improvements were primary reasons for elimination of smallpox as well as cholera and typhoid fever. For instance, he notes, no one would ever consider that vaccinations cured cholera. Yet, this scourge that previously struck every few years, killing thousands, is now virtually extinct—without vaccinations. He continues that there is always some opportunist who only wishes he would have made up and administered a vaccine simultaneous to the time of cholera's, or some other communicable disease's, elimination. Then, he would have taken credit for "stamping out" this disease too, thereby creating a future source of revenue for the medical profession. Based upon Dr. Greer's vast experience he makes a rather profound statement, that is that "vaccination does not give the least protection against smallpox, but on the contrary it increases the liability."

This is perhaps why the powers of home remedies and natural cures are rarely discussed in government circles. The federal government is under extreme financial distress. Thus, it is beholden to the financial concerns of those in power and readily bows to the interests of the few. Public interest is rarely if ever the motive. While it is true that the World Health Organization may have initially saved lives through its vaccination program, the chronic ill effects of vaccines has never been thoroughly evaluated. Perhaps the rapid death rate in Africa, where hundreds of thousands die daily from AIDS and other viral syndromes, is due to the previous and current mass vaccinations of a population which was unable to tolerate the introduction of such a vast amount of microbially contaminated injections. Future research is needed to document this possibility. However, in the future the safety of vaccines should be carefully assessed before they are administered.

There is a science to protecting the body from ill effects of vaccinations. This is the science of immune protection and immune stimulation. Vitamins which bolster immunity, such as vitamin C, vitamin B-6, pantothenic acid, and vitamin A, protect the body from the toxic effects of vaccinations. What's more, such vitamins, if well supplied in the cells, may prevent the occurrence of smallpox and similar diseases. This again illustrates the flaw of relying upon mass vaccination exclusively. Nutritional education and, thus, the regular intake of the appropriate nutrients greatly "immunizes" the body from communicable diseases. The regular intake of the aforementioned vitamins could prevent the need for mass vacination. Yet, at a minimum if you are forced to undergo a new vaccine, especially if you are an individual, you must take immune bolstering nutrients. The most important of these are vitamin C, vitamin A, pyridoxine, and selenium.

Certain herbal medicines offer potent support in reversing vaccine toxicity. Wild oregano is the most powerful of these. As a protection take a few drops of oil of P73 wild oregano under the tongue after any vaccination. Also, take Oregamax, 2 or 3 capsules twice daily. This is known as the "cleansing herb" of the ancient law, that is of the Old Testament. Thus, it can be relied upon to purge or detoxify unwanted residues.

Before synthesized drugs became established it was known that dietary and herbal therapy aided the treatment and prevention of smallpox. It was discovered that adding fresh milk to the diet resulted in a rapid improvement. This is probably because milk is rich in key vitamins, like riboflavin, vitamin A, and vitamin D, which are difficult to procure in other foods. It is also an excellent source of amino acids, so direly needed for immune health. Spearmint and peppermint teas were was used for gastric or abdominal symptoms. Honey with sage tea was used as a gargle for irritated mouth or throat. Peruvian bark was administered for the severe exhaustion. A tea made from the old southern remedy, sassafras bark plus catnip, was used to accelerate the eruptions so they would heal more quickly. According to Gunn's *Family Physician and Home Book of Health* black cohosh, also known as native rattle root, was "an important remedy in smallpox." The patient was given it regularly from the time of the first eruption until healing began. According to the editors it keeps the eruption from invading the deep tissues and causes it to be purged out of the skin. A native root compound is now available. Called SpiritDrops it is a potent root extract for regenerating and healing the body. Useful for a wide range of conditions, it would be an invaluable aid in the reversal and/or prevention of smallpox.

According to *Vitalogy,* a book written in 1930 by E. H. Ruddin, M.D., the Paris Academy of Medicine described a herbal tonic that was nearly always curative. The main ingredient was the herb foxglove, the same one from which digitalis is made. Tartaric acid, the main acidic compound in grapes and grape extracts, was regarded by English nurses as a significant cure. American nurses used a different acid, vinegar water, to sooth facial and head lesions. Smallpox was known to infect the eyes, causing blindness. Dr. Ruddin describes the frequent use of rose water essence to prevent eye infection/damage.

Treatment protocol

Use the P73 oil of wild oregano aggressively. Take it under the tongue, a few drops every hour or even every half hour. If respiratory symptoms develop, take Oregacyn, two or more capsules several times daily. Use the oil topically on any region. Also, use Skin Clenz, applying it as often as needed. For further immune support take Oregamax, three capsules three times daily. Eat large quantities of onions and garlic, as the sulfur in them helps kill germs, plus it speeds the healing of skin. Take organic selenium, 600 mcg daily, vitamin A, 10,000 I.U. daily, and vitamin C, 1000 mg twice daily. Also, take a crude natural vitamin C/flavonoid supplement, since crude natural vitamin C speeds the healing of tissues and is retained superiorly in the body, for instance, Flavin-C, three capsules every two hours. To eradicate the prostration and weakness take Royal Kick (premium-grade royal jelly), three capsules every few hours. Get a diffuser and add essential oils, like oils of lavender, neroli, rosemary, oregano, sage, etc., and disseminate throughout the air. Also, use Germ-A-Clenz. Spray it throughout the house. Spray it on furnace or air conditioning filters. Pump-spray it about the bedroom at bedtime.

Smoke inhalation

This disaster happens to thousands of North Americans daily. High levels of smoke poison the lungs, causing severe tissue damage. However, the damage caused by cigarettes is far more common and significant than disaster-related smoke damage.

Cigarette smoke causes significant tissue damage. Second-hand smoke is nearly as dangerous as actual smoking. Toxic hydrocarbons enter the lungs, causing inflammation and irritation. These hydrocarbons are among the most potent carcinogens known. One of these, nitrosamine, is so toxic that the amount of this chemical that would fit on the tip of a pin is enough to induce cancer. Yet, there are thousands of chemicals in smoke, including nitrosamines, and all of them are toxic.

Smoke can rapidly damage the lungs. However, with the use of natural medicines much of the damage can be reversed. The lungs are in dire need of antioxidants in order to cleanse themselves of toxins. Otherwise, the toxins accumulate, poisoning the outer as well as the inner parts of the lung cells. The natural antioxidants, vitamins, minerals, enzymes, and spice extracts, act as biological cleansing agents, empowering the white blood cells and other cellular aid workers in their efforts to remove accumulated poisons. The intake of these antioxidants and edible spice oils makes an enormous impact on the rate of healing of lung tissue. The edible spice oils are so effective that they can be used in the midst of a crisis to prevent severe disease and/or fatality.

Treatment protocol

To reverse the toxicity of acute exposure take Oregacyn, 2 or more capsules as needed. For an accute crisis take a capsule or 2 as often as every hour. Also, take oil of wild Oreganol, a few drops under the tongue several times daily. Rosemary, oregano, and juniper oils are invaluable antidotes to smoke, plus they are potent antioxidants. These are all found in Respira Clenz: take 10 or more drops three time daily. During an acute attack use it more aggressively, like every few minutes. Take also 10 or more drops of edible oil of rosemary in an olive oil base two times daily or as needed. While vitamins A, C, E, and beta carotene are crucial for smoke detoxification, spice extracts are far more powerful. The Oregacyn, Oreganol, and oil of Rosemary are aggressive in reversing smoke-induced lung damage. Also, the mineral selenium is an aggressive smoke antagonist: take 400 to 600 mcg of organically bound selenium daily. For acute smoke toxicity take more, for instance, 400 mcg two or three times daily. High doses of selenium can only be taken for a short period, like a few weeks. A safe daily dose is 200 to 400 mcg.

Tonsillitis

The tonsils are one of the most critical immunological organs, perhaps the most critical of all. They are the guardians to the gate of entry: the oral, digestive, and respiratory cavities. Their role is to help the body capture toxic invaders, especially germs.

It is a travesty that the usefulness of these glands has been disregarded. For decades physicians regarded them to be of no significance and, thus, frequently prescribed their removal. However, now it is known that the tonsils serve a critical function and that they should only be removed as a last resort. In fact, every effort must be made to retain them and, thus, to cure tonsular illnesses with non-surgical therapies.

For decades both doctors and patients regarded the tonsils as useless. In fact, they regarded them as disease breeding. A surgical crusade was begun in the 1950s to remove them routinely. During the height of this folly in the United States and Canada as many as 2.5 million people per year, mostly children, had their tonsils surgically removed. Thus, the crusade was largely financially motivated. Yet, the *Journal of the American Medical Association,* the most orthodox of all medical journals, claims that "Tonsils...are protective organs and should not be removed."

The tonsils are simply a mass of lymph tissue. They are rather large in childhood, when they are needed the most, and gradually shrink with age. In the elderly they are tiny but are often still functional. They should not be removed with the exception of life threatening illnesses.

The tonsils have an excellent blood supply, needed to deliver white blood cells and extract toxins. Naturally, as a result of their functions they may become inflammed and swollen. They are just performing their role of cleansing and detoxifying poisons and microbes. This swelling and pain are also a normal consequence and, other than the discomfort, are no cause for alarm. These glands do the job for which they were created: trapping and draining off infection and helping to prepare the immune system for future assaults. The tonsils are the human body's most important sentries: guarding the gate to health. Their removal greatly impairs immunity and increases the risks for chronic and serious diseases, particularly fungal infections, chronic bacterial infections, intestinal disorders and even cancer.

Swollen or sore tonsils act as a warning of infection elsewhere in the body, for instance, the teeth, sinuses, digestive tract, or lungs. They are a miraculous organ, because of their ability to warn of potential problems as well as help prevent future illnesses. One article reports that if infected teeth or sinuses are cured, tonsillar function returns to normal. Thus, removing the tonsils fails to treat the cause: chronic infection hidden somewhere in the body.

Modern medicine has basically failed to correctly treat individuals with tonsil and adenoid infections. Millions of tonsils are removed merely on the supposition that colds and sore throats would be lessened. A study of nearly 4500 children proved that removal of tonsils failed to reduce the incidence of any type of respiratory disease, including colds, ear infections, and bronchitis. The fact is there was a slight increase above normal in those whose tonsils were removed.

Treatment protocol

The tonsils are readily cleansed through the intake of potent natural antiseptics. Take oil of wild Oreganol, five to ten drops twice daily under the tongue. For severe cases take the oil several times daily, like five drops every hour or two. The Oregacyn is extremely aggressive and may be needed to help shrink the tonsillar swelling and eradicate deep-seated infections.

If infected teeth are suspected as a source for the infection, rub P73 oil of wild oregano on the involved region(s) once or twice daily. Add a drop or two of the oil to a toothbrush and brush gently. For sinus disorders take Oregacyn, one or two capsules twice daily. Continue this amount for at least two months. Also, take oil of wild oregano, 3 to 5 drops under the tongue twice daily.

Tuberculosis

This is one of the most devastating of all diseases. Incredibly, it afflicts as much as one third of the human race. In the United States it is gradually increasing in incidence, soon to again become a devastating epidemic.

The disease is caused by a germ known medically as *Mycobacterium tuberculosis*, apparently a type of bacteria. There is some doubt about this, however, as this bizarre, destructive, slow growing germ somewhat resembles a fungus. According to the editors of the *Introduction to Respiratory Diseases*, National Tuberculosis and Respiratory Disease Association, the tuberculosis germ may be regarded as sort of a fungus-bacteria. This may explain the insidious nature of this infection. It also explains the relative resistance of the germ to standard antibiotic therapy. In the earlier 1900s when millions of Americans were afflicted tuberculosis was known as consumption, because it literally consumed the individual, gradually destroying the vital tissues. Most people regard tuberculosis as only a lung disease but, in fact, it greatly and negatively affects the entire body. With time the disease causes the decay of all of the organs, even the bones, leaving the individual weakened and debilitated.

Unfortunately, tuberculosis is making a rather massive comeback. In the United States it is endemic in certain hospitals, especially those with large populations of AIDS patients. Even relatively healthy individuals are developing the disease. Vegetarians are at a high risk, because a lack of high grade protein diminishes immunity. Plus, complete avoidance of animal foods causes stomach atrophy. Such damage to the stomach halts the production of stomach acid, needed to sterilize food. Thus, if tubercular germs are ingested, they gain entrance to the blood and/or organs, causing infection.

Tuberculosis is readily spread on airlines. The air filters in the jets/planes may become contaminated. If air is stagnant or if filters spew the germs, virtually anyone on the plane may become infected. This is perhaps the most common mode of inoculation. Hundreds, rather, thousands, of flight attendants have become infected in this manner, and most of them have yet to be diagnosed. This is because it may take several years for the symptoms of tuberculosis to manifest.

The tuberculosis germ readily hides. Its main site may not be the lungs: it may be the teeth or sinuses—even the kidneys. Thus, excellent oral hygiene as well as proper health of the sinuses, perhaps through regular sinus gavage, may be necessary to eradicate and/or prevent this illness.

Treatment protocol

Tuberculosis is one of the most difficult of all illnesses to cure. It is chronic, which means that it is a slow growing, that is smoldering infection, which is difficult to eradicate. The unassisted immune system often fails to cure it. However, antiseptic spice extracts offer hope for a cure.

The key is to take the supplements regularly; never miss a dose. This is essential, because it is critical to maintain proper blood levels of the antiseptic to eradicate this infection. This is a chronic and significant disease: it is nothing to take lightly. It requires a monumental effort to cure, and consistency is the key. As the most powerful natural antiseptic available, take Oregacyn, 3 capsules twice daily. Tougher cases may require massive doses, for instance, 5 capsules three times daily. Take also SuperStrength oil of wild oregano, 20 drops under the tongue twice daily. For difficult cases take more, like 20 to 40 drops three times daily. Get as much sunlight as possible. If you must spend much of your time indoors, buy full spectrum lights, and install them in all fixtures/lamps. Keep windows open as much as possible. Eat large amounts of high protein food. If you can tolerate it, drink a quart of whole organic milk daily. Follow the diet in Dr. Cass Ingram's *How to Eat Right and Live Longer*. Take a natural vitamin C supplement, such as Potent-C and/or Flavin-C, about 200 mg of natural vitamin C daily (follow the label claims on the bottles to know the amount to take).

For excellent sinus health do a daily sinus gavage. Snort saline water into the nostrils two or three times daily. Press one nostril closed, and inhale the saline water with the other; allow the fluid to either come out through the mouth or back through the nostrils. Also, oil of wild oregano and oil of wild bay leaf are excellent for sinus cleansing. Place a drop or two in the salt water. Or, take a few drops under the tongue twice daily.

Multiple spice extracts offer the greatest hope for a cure. Drugs are largely impotent, plus they exhibit numerous side effects. Blindness is a common side effect of anti-tuberculosis drugs. Spice extracts have been shown to kill TB germs. The fact is they are capable of sterilizing sewage. These heat-producing extracts are among the most powerful germ killing substances known, and, since they are from edible plants, they are far safer than other medicinal herbs and certainly infinitely safer than drugs. As immunity tonics these extracts are extremely beneficial for TB patients. As a result of their regular use, usually energy, strength, and lung function improve within days.

Valley fever (Coccidiomycoses)

This is a desert or southwestern infection caused by the fungus Coccidiodes immitis. It only exists in certain parts of southern California, Arizona, New Mexico, and Texas. Mexico is another hotbed for this infection. It is usually not found in northern Texas. This fungus thrives only in hot dry regions, and its spores exist on dust or dry vegetation. It is carried mainly by rodents. The main area it attacks is the lungs.

Millions of individuals living in the Southwest may unknowingly contract this disease. In other words there may be millions of asymptomatic carriers. When it attacks, it may commonly be confused with the flu. It develops from inhaling dust which contains the spores. Inhaling spores may not immediately result in active infection. It may strike later if the individual is under stress or suffers from diminished immunity. However, if a symptomatic infection occurs, it develops about one to two weeks after inhaling the dust. Respiratory symptoms are the main feature, but in a small percentage skin lesions and joint pain develop. Thus, an individual who visits the Southwest and later, for instance, within a month of two, becomes deathly ill may well have developed coccidiodes infection.

Treatment protocol

Oregacyn is a potent nutritional supplement for this condition. Take two capsules twice daily. Also, take P73 oil of wild oregano, five to ten drops twice daily. Also, to improve blood flow in the lungs, take edible oil of rosemary, 10 drops twice daily. Respira Clenz is also a potent extract for the lungs. Take 10 drops twice daily.

Whooping cough

This is an infection which afflicts the throat, bronchial tubes, and lungs. It is characterized by bizarre bouts of coughing, with a whoop-like sound. The disease is caused by a bacteria known as *Bordetella pertussis*, which is why the disease is also known as pertussis.

Pertussis is easily spread and usually occurs in children, although adults are far from immune. Americans are immunized against pertussis, however, outbreaks are occurring even in immunized individuals.

Symptoms usually begin as a cold-like syndrome, followed in a few days by a cough that is a series of short, quick coughs succeeded by a whooping-like noise, that is a long drawn out crowing sound. This "whoop" is caused by deep inspiration while the vocal cords are tightened. This is usually repeated several times, and the attack often ends with the expulsion of thick or sticky mucus. It may also end with vomiting, which occurs because of the tremendous pressure of the cough. The disease is curable and is rarely fatal. While extremely rare, serious complications may occur, like pneumonia. However, hospitalization, largely out of fear, is common.

Treatment protocol

Potent spice extracts are the ideal natural tonic for this illness. Take Oregacyn, one or two capsules three times daily. During an attack open the capsule and place a quarter teaspoon of the powder under the tongue. Let this melt, and repeat every 15 minutes or so. Be sure to keep the room of the sufferer well ventilated. Also, take P73 oil of wild oregano, two or more drops under the tongue several times daily. This alone should eliminate the cough. In infants simply rub the oil on the feet or chest; it isn't necessary to give it internally.

Chapter 5

Staying Healthy

Today, it is a challenge to stay healthy. From the point of view of overall health this is perhaps the most dangerous time ever in history. In general medical science is doing a poor job of helping people stay healthy and an even poorer job of helping them cure their chronic diseases. For instance, the majority of chronic diseases, such as cancer, diabetes, high blood pressure, heart disease, lupus, arthritis, fibromyalgia, chronic fatigue syndrome, asthma, and numerous others, are increasing in incidence, not decreasing.

It takes effort to maintain strong health. Yet, this is perhaps the most critical effort anyone can make. This is because the health of the body is the basis of all activity, productivity, inventiveness, and even spirituality.

The power of systematic exercise

Exercise is a powerful and effective medicine for the lungs. A lack of exercise leads to lung congestion and, thus, the accumulation of toxins.

Systematic exercise is the ideal type for lung health. This means adhering to a routine. However, it is unnecessary to perform heavy exercise. A simple one or two mile walk, if done regularly, is sufficient. So is regular swimming or bicycling. Jogging is acceptable, if it is done on soft surfaces and if it is away from heavily polluted regions, like busy road sides. However, walking is by far the ideal lung-healthy exercise. This is because it is highly relaxing, and, thus, it allows time for deep breathing. It also allows for enjoyment of beautiful countryside, which is relaxing to the central nervous system. It is the central nervous system which controls breathing. It is critical for the nervous system to be healthy and relaxed in order for the lungs to be as healthy as possible.

Improved posture

Poor posture has particularly derogatory effects upon lung function. The lungs are closely connected to the spine. Any alteration in position or disruption in spinal anatomy negatively affects them.

Check your posture frequently. Look in the mirror. Are you hunched over? Are you constantly slouching? Is your back excessively bowed? All of these abnormal positions greatly impede lung function. If this postural dysfunction is prolonged, dysfunction, as well as disease, will develop.

Improving the posture often results in an immediate improvement of health. If the posture has been poor for a prolonged period, postural exercise may be required. Proper chiropractic or osteopathic care often results in improved posture.

Deep breathing

Improved posture and deep breathing are directly connected. If the posture is poor, it is impossible to breathe normally and deeply. Carefully watch your posture by reviewing your standing and sitting postures in a mirror daily. Make a conscious effort to correct any imbalances. Keep your spine erect and pull in your abdomen.

Start your deep breathing program right away. You can do it on your own. Take a deep breath and exhale slowly. Repeatedly taking deep breaths will force you to stand and sit taller. It is impossible to take deep breaths if you are in a slouched position. This deep breathing will stretch the rib cage, which will ultimately help improve both your sitting and standing postures.

You must make an effort to breathe correctly. Relax your abdominal muscles. Do relaxing exercises, like gentle stretching or body shaking. Loosen up. Being uptight is the greatest reason for restricted breathing. Once you relax, you can breathe fully and deeply. Breathe in to the count of four. Hold the breath for the count of four, then exhale slowly over the count of four. Do this exercise as often as possible as three repetitions of the entire technique throughout the day. This deep breathing technique is described by the book *Smoke Enders* and is used successfully for aborting cigarette addiction.

Proper ventilation

For the purposes of human health this means the movement of fresh air through indoor facilities. Stagnant air inside of buildings is a major cause of human disease. Incredibly, there is actually a science to the proper flow of air inside of buildings, one that is rarely taken into account when modern buildings are built. The editors of the *Modern Home Physician*, published in

1947, describe this dilemma thusly: "If...access of air to dwellings is prevented by their being crowded together or anything prevents its passage through the dwellings, *ill health is bound to follow* (italics mine)." In other words, air must constantly circulate. Stale or stagnant air concentrates toxic fumes and microbes, which, when inhaled, lead to illness.

Many people are concerned about opening windows, because they feel they are sensitive to a draught. They might believe the draught would cause them to become ill, for instance, to catch cold. There may be some truth to this concern. However, proper ventilation prevents this. The correct method to ventilate is to open one or more windows widely. Opening windows partially causes draughts, which forces the air in at an abnormal rate. In other words, the rapid movement of the air is what causes the chill, not the cold air itself. Thus, if two or more windows are opened widely in the facility, draughts are prevented. In other words open the storm doors completely, not just a mere slit. Don't open a door partially; open it widely. This will help solve problems of air sensitivity and/or chilling.

Adrenal weakness: its role in respiratory disorders

The adrenal glands play an instrumental role in respiratory health. They are the main defense against allergy and toxic chemical inhalation. They also help maintain normal blood flow, which is crucial for proper oxygen delivery. If the strength of the adrenals fails, so fails the health of the lungs.

The adrenal glands are essential for fighting allergic reactions. They produce the natural steroids needed to ward off irritations and inflammation. These steroids include natural cortisone, which is a potent antiinflammatory agent.

There are a number of causes for reduced adrenal gland function. Stress greatly depletes these glands. So does poor nutrition. A high intake of sugar causes the depletion of cortisone reserves. Alcohol also destroys cortisone.

Boosting adrenal function greatly improves the body's ability to withstand the everyday stress of daily living. This benefit is also of great value with asthma, which is a stress response indicating poor adrenal reserve. By building up the adrenal capacity, the asthma gradually improves. The role of the adrenals is so profound that virtually any lung condition will benefit from improving their function: even emphysema and lung cancer.

Certain nutritional supplements and/or herbs may help enhance adrenal function. Perhaps the most powerful of all is royal jelly. This is because royal jelly is a type of natural steroid source. In fact, this bee product contains as many as 55 different natural steroids. The steroids in royal jelly are non-toxic.

A natural and fortified royal jelly is available. Called Royal Kick, it is a stabilized and fortified royal jelly of high potency. Fortified with extra pantothenic acid and crude natural vitamin C, this is a particularly potent formula. In my experience this formula is far superior to the commercial types in terms of the clinical response seen in patients.

How to strengthen the adrenal glands

The function of these glands can be greatly boosted. Certain vitamins are needed for adrenal steroid synthesis. The main ones are vitamins A, the B vitamin pantothenic acid, and vitamin C. To increase the strength of these glands take a natural vitamin A source, like cod liver oil, about a half teaspoon daily (Note: infants or children should not take this amount). Also, take a natural vitamin C source, like Flavin-C or Potent-C, about 200 mg daily. Royal jelly is a superb tonic for the adrenals. This is because this substance contains up to 55 different adrenal hormones and it is easy to digest and absorb. Plus, in contrast to synthetic cortisone/steroids, it is completely nontoxic. Take a crude high grade royal jelly capsule, such as Royal Kick, about 4 to 6 capsules in the a.m. daily. The latter contains some pantothenic acid, about 100 mg per capsule. In certain cases mega doses of pantothenic acid may be needed. I have prescribed as much as 1000 mg of a powdered pantothenic acid capsule two or three times daily as a natural means to bolster cortisone production. This vitamin is free of significant side effects, although high doses could cause loose stools. The fact is high dose pantothenic acid is an excellent remedy for constipation.

Drug toxicity: a cause of respiratory symptoms

In order to keep the respiratory system as healthy as possible, it is crucial to avoid the use of drugs. Numerous drugs may induce respiratory symptoms. In fact, many are outright respiratory poisons. Thus, a lung, sinus, or bronchial condition may develop strictly as a drug side effect. Cough, especially a dry type, is perhaps the most common type. High blood pressure drugs commonly cause this, particularly the so called ACE inhibitors. Recently, it was found that the dry cough caused by these drugs is somehow related to iron deficiency. Giving iron reverses the cough. Thus, if you are taking medications and suddenly develop respiratory symptoms, see your doctor about reducing the dosage or, preferably, eliminating the drugs.

Keep the air healthy: the powers of Germ-A-Clenz

Germ-A-Clenz is a special solution of essential oils for cleansing the air. It is highly useful for making home or work safe by keeping the air as "microbially purified" as possible. It does so without chemicals: only pure unprocessed essential oils are used, thus it enhances air quality.

The majority of commercially available essential oil-based "air purifiers" are fraudulent. They contain synthetic chemicals as well as chemically processed essential oils.

Germ-A-Clenz is exceptionally useful for cleansing the air and preventing respiratory infections. Its value is obvious during the winter and summer when indoor air can become stagnant. Simply spray this wonderfully aromatic spray into the air once or twice daily, or add a few drops of Germ-A-Clenz to a humidifier or vaporizer. Spray furnace/air conditioner filters frequently to decrease mold and viral transmission. Also, spray it around vents or any other region where air flows. Spray the air in restrooms, the hotbed for germs, on a regular basis. Today, largely due to global warming, there is a mold and fungus epidemic. Germ-A-Clenz can control or eliminate this problem. Germ-A-Clenz is available in two forms: a spray bottle and a two ounce dropper bottle.

We live in a highly toxic, polluted world. The air is fouled, and so is our food. While our options are rather limited, we should not give up hope. There are answers, and those answers are found in nature.

Spice extracts, such as Oreganol and Oregacyn, offer

tremendous hope and value for victims of lung and respiratory disorders. Modern medicine offers little or no hope, especially for individuals with chronic diseases. What's more, many of the medical therapies exhibit significant side effects. Furthermore, drugs never cure chronic respiratory conditions. There are no serious side effects from the use of properly produced, natural spice extracts. The only issue is that in large doses it may be necessary to also take healthy bacteria, since any germicide is capable of killing healthy as well as pathogenic bacteria. Even so, spices are foods and, therefore, they are completely edible. Long used as medicines, they are far safer than drugs as well as medicinal non-edible herbs such as goldenseal, ginseng, and gotu kola. Plus, in contrast to many over-the-counter respiratory medicines and weak commercial herbs, spice extracts are highly effective. Results are often noticed in minutes. If you are skeptical, you may end up sick a lot longer than you need to be. These extracts are potent germicides, and they don't discriminate: they kill every germ known to humankind. Use them to help reverse your respiratory condition(s). Take them to bolster overall health. Take advantage of these gifts of almighty God. Your life may depend upon it.

Chapter 6

Conclusion

The respiratory system is the most vulnerable of all systems to germ or toxic invasions. It represents direct access to the internal and potentially vulnerable tissues. A mere breath can give life, but it can also bring disease—even death.

The health of the respiratory system is dependent upon numerous factors: healthy lifestyle, proper diet, proper hygiene, and, of course, clean air. While the latter may be difficult to achieve, air can be cleansed, through the appropriate filters and purifiers.

Invariably, the lungs and other respiratory organs need significant biological and chemical support to remain in optimal health. Air pollution greatly damages them, lowering their resistance to disease. Attempts must be made to keep the lungs in as clean of a condition as possible. This cannot be achieved with proper diet and exercise alone. Nutritional supplements and detoxification—that is the use of natural compounds to bolster respiratory health and clean out toxins—this is the approach that will produce predictable, positive results. Vitamins, minerals, antioxidants, herbal extracts, spice extracts, and medicinal foods, like honey and vinegar, are powerful tools for regenerating the lungs and keeping them as healthy as possible.

Today, we live in an incredibly toxic world. Adding to the toxicity by taking harsh drugs is bound to diminish lung health. The effort should be to reduce the intake of harsh medications, relying on the more gentle, yet, powerful, natural medicines, which will not cause organ toxicity.

This is why nutritional supplements are the answer for enhancing respiratory health. They strengthen the lungs. They help cleanse the sinuses. They purge poisons from the tonsils. They keep the lung and sinus passages open. Plus, they aid the body in the removal of poisons and in the destruction of germs. What's more, there are natural agents which are germicidal which are of enormous value. This is because they destroy germs virtually on contact, which is of lifesaving value for respiratory conditions. The fact is the daily intake of natural antiseptics can help overall health dramatically by curtailing the incidence of respiratory infections.

Prevention is the key for maintaining a strong, healthy body. Respiratory infections can be dangerous, and there may be no guarantee that the infection can be cured, especially if treatment begins too late. However, in general the natural antiseptics are so powerful, so valuable, that they will help virtually at any stage in the infection. This is because these antiseptics are capable of killing in minutes: in fact, seconds. Thus, a thorough knowledge of what is needed for such protection is crucial in order to prevent serious illness.

Spice extracts offer germicidal power unknown in the drug kingdom. Furthermore, spices are well respected for their diversity of effects upon the respiratory system. They aid in keeping the respiratory passages open, decreasing mucous or thinning it. They help neutralize the toxicity of allergens. Thus, their actions cover the gamut of needs for reversing respiratory illnesses.

Plagues will happen. Chronic types of "plague" already exist. If used systematically, the information in this book could save thousands, perhaps millions, of lives. Plus, it could give life to the already living.

Appendix

Foods or Food Additives that May Act as Respiratory Poisons

- food dyes
- refined sugar
- nitrated/processed meats
- wheat or wheat germ
- cow's milk
- peanuts and peanut butter
- baker's and brewer's yeast
- chocolate
- eggs
- soy
- malt and barley
- seafood (especially lobster, shrimp, crab, sole, flounder, and crab)

Foods or Food Additives Likely to Cause Sinus Problems

- aspartame
- yellow dye # 5 (tartrazine)
- butter
- wheat and wheat germ
- peanuts and peanut butter
- eggs

- cheese
- chocolate
- cream
- cow's milk
- fruit drinks
- soda pop
- refined sugar
- citrus juice (in some instances, especially the highly processed types)

Foods which Enhance Respiratory Functions

- rosemary
- oregano
- ginger
- caraway
- cumin
- mustard
- basil
- sage
- thyme
- pumpkin seeds and pumpkinseed oil (as a source of natural fatty acids, zinc (in the seeds), and phospholipids
- fresh citrus juice (as a rich source of vitamin C)
- spinach
- radishes

- wasabi
- broccoli
- egg yolks (as a source of phospholipids)
- garlic
- onion
- beef broth
- chicken broth
- nuts and seeds
- fresh red meat (as a source of amino acids and phospholipids)
- organic liver (as a source of vitamin A and phospholipids)
- pumpkin and squash (as a source of vitamin A in the form of beta carotene)
- sweet potatoes (as a source of vitamin A in the form of beta carotene)
- horseradish and salmon (as a source of fatty fish oils and phospholipids, as well as animal-source vitamin A)
- herring and sardines (as a source of fatty fish oils and vitamin A) cheddar and Swiss cheese

- hot chili peppers
- parsley (as a source of magnesium)
- beet and turnip greens (as a source of vitamin A in the form of beta carotene)

- nettles

- dandelion

- rose hips

Foods or Food Additives Likely to Provoke Asthma Attacks

- yellow dye # 5 (tartrazine)

- baker's and brewer's yeast

- cow's milk

- wheat

- malt or barley

- corn

- red wine

- refined sugar......refined vegetable oils

- brominated vegetable oils

- hydrogenated vegetable oils

- partially hydrogenated vegetable oils

- lard

- cottonseed meal or oil

- MSG

Bibliography

Anderson, W. A. D. 1960. *Synopsis of Pathology*. St. Louis: C. V. Mosby Co.

Birkeland, Jorgen. 1949. *Microbiology and Man*. New York: Appleton-Century-Crofts.

Evans, W. A. 1917. *How to Keep Well*. New York: D. Appelton and Co.

The Editors. *Our Human Body*. Pleasantville, NY: Reader's Digest.

Fishbein, M. 1956. *Modern Home Medical Adviser*. New York: Garden City Books.

Haas, F. and S. Haas.1990. *The Chronic Bronchitis and Emphysema Handbook*. New York: John Wiley & Sons.

Harris, A. and M. Super. 1995. *Cystic Fibrosis: the Facts*. Oxford: Oxford Univ. Press.

Introduction to Respiratory Diseases. 1969. National Tuberculosis and Respiratory Disease Association.

Lindlar, V. H. 1943. *Most Popular Foreign Dishes*. New York: Journal of Living Publ.

Lorand, A. 1928. *Health Through Rational Diet*. Philadelphia: F. A. Davis Co.

Fishbein, M. 1970. *Medical and Health Encyclopedia: V.* 18. New York: H. S. Stuttman Co.

Robinson, V. 1947. *The New Modern Home Physician*. New York: Wm. Wise & Co.

Seltzer, A. 1949. *Your Nasal Sinuses and Their Disorders*. New York: Froben Press.

Smith, W.H. 1884. *The Human Body and Its Health*. New York: American Book Co.

Weinstein, A. 1987. *Asthma*. St. Louis: McGraw-Hill.

Index